Return to *The House of God*

Literature and Medicine

MARTIN KOHN AND CAROL DONLEY, EDITORS

1 *Literature and Aging: An Anthology*
   EDITED BY MARTIN KOHN, CAROL DONLEY, AND DELESE WEAR

2 *The Tyranny of the Normal: An Anthology*
   EDITED BY CAROL DONLEY AND SHERYL BUCKLEY

3 *What's Normal? Narratives of Mental and Emotional Disorders*
   EDITED BY CAROL DONLEY AND SHERYL BUCKLEY

4 *Recognitions: Doctors and Their Stories*
   EDITED BY CAROL DONLEY AND MARTIN KOHN

5 *Chekhov's Doctors: A Collection of Chekhov's Medical Tales*
   EDITED BY JACK COULEHAN

6 *Tenderly Lift Me: Nurses Honored, Celebrated, and Remembered*
   BY JEANNE BRYNER

7 *The Poetry of Nursing: Poems and Commentaries of Leading Nurse-Poets*
   EDITED BY JUDY SCHAEFER

8 *Our Human Hearts: A Medical and Cultural Journey*
   BY ALBERT HOWARD CARTER III

9 *Fourteen Stories: Doctors, Patients, and Other Strangers*
   BY JAY BARUCH

10 *Stories of Illness and Healing: Women Write Their Bodies*
   EDITED BY SAYANTANI DASGUPTA AND MARSHA HURST

11 *Wider than the Sky: Essays and Meditations on the Healing Power of Emily Dickinson*
   EDITED BY CINDY MACKENZIE AND BARBARA DANA

12 *Lisa's Story: The Other Shoe*
   BY TOM BATIUK

13 *Bodies and Barriers: Dramas of Dis-Ease*
   EDITED BY ANGELA BELLI

14 *The Spirit of the Place: A Novel*
   BY SAMUEL SHEM

15 *Return to The House of God: Medical Resident Education 1978–2008*
   EDITED BY MARTIN KOHN AND CAROL DONLEY

Return to
The House of God

༄

Medical Resident Education
1978–2008

༄

Edited by Martin Kohn

& Carol Donley

༄

The Kent State

University Press

KENT, OHIO

༄

© 2008 by The Kent State University Press, Kent, Ohio 44242

ALL RIGHTS RESERVED

Library of Congress Catalog Card Number 2008021131

ISBN 978-0-87338-983-9

Manufactured in the United States of America

"Mayhem at the Hospital" is from *More Matter: Essays and Criticism*
by John Updike, copyright © 1999 by John Updike.
Used by permission of Alfred A. Knopf, a division of Random House, Inc.

The following poems are reprinted by permission of the publisher:
"Foley" by Mindy Shah, "He Still Whistles" by Jerald Winakur,
"Intensive Care" by Mindy Shah, "January Thaw" by Richard Berlin,
"NG Tube" by Sarah Jane Cook, "October 1st" by Mairi Leining,
"On Call, 3 A.M." by Richard Berlin, and "Pandora" by Kelley Jean White from *Body Language*,
copyright © 2006 by Neeta Jain, Dagan Coppock, and Stephanie Brown Clark,
BOA Editions, Ltd., www.boaeditions.org.

LIBRARY OF CONGRESS CATALOGING-IN-PUBLICATION DATA

Return to The house of God : medical resident education, 1978–2008 /
edited by Martin Kohn and Carol Donley.
p.   cm. — (Literature and medicine ; 15)
Includes bibliographical references.
ISBN 978-0-87338-983-9 (pbk. : alk. paper) ∞
1. Shem, Samuel. House of God.   2. Shem, Samuel—Influence.
3. Residents (Medicine)—United States.
4. Literature and medicine—United States—History—20th century.
I. Kohn, Martin. II. Donley, Carol C.
PS3569.H39374H6837 2008
813'.54—dc22
2008021131

British Library Cataloging-in-Publication data are available.

12 11 10 09 08   5 4 3 2 1

To my wife and children—thanks as always for your love and support. MK

To my husband and children. You're the best. CD

Contents

∾

Introduction
    MARTIN KOHN AND CAROL DONLEY   xi
The Birth of The House of God
    DENIS NOBLE   1

Residency Education in Historical Perspective

Houses of God before Shem: Boston City and the Thorndike
at Bellevue
    GERALD WEISSMANN   11
Residency Education since The House of God
    KENNETH M. LUDMERER   22
From The House of God *to the House of Siemens:*
Bedside Skills Thirty Years Later
    SARAH LAPEY, JUDY MCCARTER, AND ABRAHAM VERGHESE   35
The Godless Kingdom: Medical Education in France, 1973–2008
    MARC ZAFFRAN (MARTIN WINCKLER)   43

Justice, Virtue, and the Laws of *The House of God*

Justice and Humor in The House of God
    MARTHA ELKS AND ISAAC M. T. MWASE   57
Wearing the Ring of Gyges in the House of God
    JULIE M. AULTMAN   74
The Laws of the House of God Revisited: or, Sneaking Primary
Care into Man's Greatest Hospital
    HOWARD BRODY   91

Literary Perspectives and Criticism

Mayhem at the Hospital
JOHN UPDIKE   103
Imagining the House of God
JACK COULEHAN   106
Writing the Medical Training Experience in 1978 and 2006:
Body Language in The House of God
STEPHANIE BROWN CLARK, NEETA JAIN, AND DAGAN COPPOCK 117
The Popocatepetl of Medicine
ARKO ODERWALD   142

Women's Perspectives and Criticism

Objects, Not Allies: Nurses in The House of God *and*
Graduate Medical Education
AMY HADDAD   153
"Fiction as Resistance": The Fat Man and the Woman Reader
ANNE HUDSON JONES   162
The Madwoman in the Attic
SUSAN ONTHANK MATES   167

Rereadings

Chasing Fire Engines
CORTNEY DAVIS   175
Speaking the Unspeakable
JAY BARUCH   182
Shem Redux: Is It Time?
STEVEN HYMAN   187
The House of God Redux
THOMAS DUFFY   190
You Gotta Know the Territory: The House of God *as Job Description*
PERRI KLASS   195
Attending in the House of God
ABIGAIL ZUGER   206

Comments from the House of Shem

Living with Shem: Reflections on the Journey of a Writer-Healer
   JANET SURREY   215
Resistance and Healing
   SAMUEL SHEM AND STEPHEN BERGMAN   221

Contributors   237

Introduction

MARTIN KOHN AND CAROL DONLEY

Every story has a beginning, and just as we've started this volume with Denis Noble's illuminating essay "The Birth of *The House of God*," what follows is an account of how this venture was born.

In late August of 2004, Brian Mandell, vice chairman of medicine for education at the Cleveland Clinic, drove the thirty or so miles from Cleveland to Hiram College to meet with us and Glenn Sharfman, associate dean of the college at that time. James Young, chairman of the Division of Medicine at the Cleveland Clinic, had asked Brian to develop a medical humanities program for the division, and according to Cleveland Clinic staff physician Yvonne Braver, wife of Hiram faculty member Lee Braver, the first place to visit would have to be the Center for Literature and Medicine.

Shortly after that meeting, a plan was devised to invite presenters to both the Cleveland Clinic campus (for grand rounds) and the Hiram College campus (as convocation speakers). At the top of the list of invitees was Stephen Bergman's name.

Steve's visit in the fall of 2005 went well. As expected, there were large audiences and lively responses to his presentations. But although our collaborative programming was in its infancy at this time, Jim Young was already yearning for something more enduring than hit-and-run visits by physician-writers and medical humanities scholars. As we mulled over Jim's suggestion, thinking about the relevance of *The House of God* to current issues in residency education, we realized we were just a few years shy of the novel's thirtieth anniversary. The idea of creating a volume of critical and reflective essays for publication in 2008, the year of *The House of God*'s thirtieth anniversary, soon was presented to all the pertinent local parties, including our editor at the Kent State University Press. And all were quite excited about the undertaking. Field testing at the fall 2005 American Society for Bioethics and Humanities annual meeting had, in fact, already indicated that there would be interest in such a project. Howard Brody, for one, was already working on a piece about the laws of the House of God, and Anne Hudson Jones was eager to lend her critical acumen to our efforts. And from an unexpected source, the *New Zealand Medical Student Journal*, we stumbled on an article titled "Medicine's Heretic Bible Nearly 30 Years Onward." In the article the author, Kit Boyes, explained, "I did do my research before entering medicine. I spoke to six doctors. The first told me I was nuts, and to buy a book called *The House of God.* The second said exactly the same, and it's been translated into 20 languages. Docs 3 through 5 checked that I'd read it. And the sixth, well I started this review with the sixth" (1). His response to imagined fellow students' queries as to whether or not they needed to read the book: "Dunno, ask me after I've been a house officer" (3). Well, we know that if it could possibly play in New Zealand, it should play well elsewhere, so return to *The House of God* we did.

We've had some fun with the title. Does it sound like the remake of a scary movie? For some it will. For others if may sound like an exhortation to read it again as a kind of penance, as a way to be reminded of what's truly important about being a doctor. What we know for sure is that *The House of God* is still alive. It has become iconic. Like all art, it gives rise to a range of emotions and makes us wonder more deeply about this world we live in, specifically the world of medical training. And for that we owe Steve Bergman our gratitude.

By mid-2006 we'd developed a list of potential contributors, some of whom we would ask to write critical essays from a variety of disciplinary vantage points addressing themes raised in the original, and others who would be asked to write reflective essays or fiction based on their reading (or rereading) of *The House of God* and then relate their contribution to their practice and/or teaching of residents. The vast majority of those we asked to contribute were not only willing but eager to do so. Our volume began to take shape over the next year and a half.

Shortly after *Return to* The House of God: *Medical Resident Education 1978–2008* began to take shape, Steve thought it might be fitting for some of the essayists, and perhaps others in medical education, to share their work at a symposium on *The House of God* in particular and medical resident education more generally. Since we'd been offering annual seminars and symposia for the past fifteen years, we slotted in for 2008 an international symposium at which this volume will be launched. We want to express our deep appreciation to the Wish, Cope & Life Foundation and to the Division of Medicine at the Cleveland Clinic for their generous support of the symposium. This volume is the fifteenth in our Literature and Medicine series, but it represents what we hope is the first of many enduring projects with our colleagues Jim Young and Brian Mandell at the Cleveland Clinic. Special thanks are due as well to Tod Chambers, past president of the American Society for Bioethics and Humanities, and to the ASBH Board for allowing us to "front end" our symposium to the 2008 annual meeting held in Cleveland, Ohio. Many thanks, too, to Marcia R. Silver for carefully reading a draft of this volume.

As we began to read the contributions that were sent to us, we found that they seemed almost to arrange themselves into clusters. We followed their lead, watching how they reinforced and sometimes contradicted each other. Oxford professor emeritus of cardiovascular physiology Denis Noble was present at the conception of *The House of God*. When his student Rhodes scholar Steve Bergman announced he was quitting science so he could write, Noble offered him a sherry. We chose Noble's essay to open the collection. He gives a remarkable critique of the dominant scientific view that pervades the modern world and medical training and contributes to the dehumanization in the novel.

The next four essays focus on historical perspectives of residency education. Gerald Weissmann looks at "Houses of God before Shem: Boston City and the Thorndike at Bellevue." Weissmann, who served as chief resident under Lewis Thomas, describes the history of the two great hospitals and his own demanding and challenging residency years, which, nevertheless, he remembers as the best of times. Internist, medical educator, and historian of medicine Kenneth M. Ludmerer writes that not only was the portrayal of medical residency accurate in *The House of God*, but most of the problems still remain. Sarah Lapey, Judy McCarter, and Abraham Verghese discuss the transition from *The House of God* to the House of Siemens, looking at bedside skills thirty years after the novel was first published. Giving us a comparison from another country, Marc Zaffran (Martin Winckler) describes "The Godless Kingdom: Medical Education in France, 1973–2008," an account that makes Roy Basch's experience seem almost benign.

Philosophical perspectives guide the next three essays. First, Morehouse professor Martha Elks and Tuskegee professor Isaac M. T. Mwase examine "Justice and Humor in *The House of God*." They note that the cynical humor of the novel is provoked by injustices throughout the system. Second, exploring virtue in the novel, Julie M. Aultman notes that "those at the top, the Slurpers, possess great power but at the same time promote injustice within the clinical setting such that cure, the only perceived goal of medicine, takes precedence over both patient *and* physician care." In the third essay, Howard Brody thoughtfully studies the Fat Man's laws, noting how they allow for "sneaking primary care into Man's Greatest Hospital." Although the laws seem to be ironic and comical, Brody points out that they actually contain much medical wisdom.

The next four essays are forms of literary criticism. In the first, we reprint John Updike's Introduction to the 1995 edition of *The House of God*. In the second essay, Jack Coulehan, professor emeritus of medicine and preventive medicine at Stony Brook University, wonders about the novel's effect on physicians-to-be in terms of its overwhelmingly cynical tone. In the third, physician, literary scholar, and historian of medicine Stephanie Brown Clark describes the development of the literature-and-medicine and medical humanities fields, which counter and complement the limitations of science as a way of understanding. In the same essay, Neeta Jain and Dagan Coppock, both recent graduates of residency programs, discuss how Bergman used the writing of the novel as a catharsis. "Thirty years later, the same forces moved us to create *Body Language*. As an exercise in catharsis, it too made the burden of human suffering and the exhaustion of medical training more bearable." In the last essay, Arko Oderwald, physician and philosopher at the Free Medical Center in Amsterdam, compares Bergman's novel about his residency in psychiatry, *Mount Misery,* with two other works: a short story called "The Psychiatrist" by Joaquim Maria Machado de Assis, a Brazilian writer; and the novel *Under the Volcano,* by Malcolm Lowry.

The next set of essays explores women's perspectives on the novel. Amy Haddad, in "Objects, Not Allies: Nurses in *The House of God* and Graduate Medical Education," argues that "Shem is not interested in drawing attention to the subservient role of nurses in health care. Nurses in *The House of God* are at best part of the background, and at worst idiotic, incompetent sex objects." Anne Hudson Jones notes that there are no positive medical women in the novel. In fact, one of the worst characters is Jo, an attending whose "do everything" creed is the exact opposite of the Fat Man's law to "do as much nothing as possible." Susan Onthank Mates presents, with biting humor and pathos, a short story about a cardiologist, Jo (based on Shem's character), who creates her own laws, such as "Medical training was hazing for boy geeks."

The last set of essays contains various rereadings of *The House of God,* in which many of the writers express different takes on the novel from those they had at first. Cortney Davis originally found the novel to be hilarious; on rereading it, she did not find it to be funny but understood that writing the novel was a way for Bergman to survive, to move to caring and healing, just as her writing allows her to do. Physician-writer Jay Baruch writes that doctoring is "an emotional contact sport" that places great demands on the brain and the heart. Medical training needs to nurture the heart as well as test the brain. Provost of Harvard University Steven Hyman found that rereading *The House of God* after many years brought back not only memories of his own residency but also visceral reactions and feelings long buried. In some ways, he thinks, today's residents have it harder than Roy Basch because of the rapid turnover in patients and the serious illnesses of those who are in the hospital. Head of the Program for Humanities and Medicine at Yale University School of Medicine Thomas Duffy reports that the feelings arising from his rereading of the book were quite different from his original disgust with it. Now he understands that "the real power and prescience of the novel are in its depiction of the unacceptable cost and casualties of some medical training." The next rereading comes from physician-author Perri Klass, who first read the book as a medical student and was immensely relieved because it explained to her why she did not go into internal medicine. Now she comments, "I reread *The House of God,* and I still feel that the take-home message is, Whatever you do, stay out of academic tertiary care internal medicine. . . . There are truths here about life and death and medicine; there are legitimate protests against an inhumane system—but there is also that sense of being in the wrong place, doing the wrong job." Like Stephen Bergman and Roy Basch, Perri Klass found a better fit for herself. In the last work in this section, Abigail Zuger tells a story of what it's like today being an attending, taking care of residents as they do their rotation in internal medicine. "Your interns have three times as many patients to care for as they should. They have so many patients they can barely talk to any of them; their days are occupied with answering pages and trying to get blood drawn and labs scheduled." And meanwhile, the hospital administration is murmuring that the patients are being kept in the hospital too long (for the bottom line).

Our final essays come from Janet Surrey and her husband, Stephen Bergman. She describes being with Bergman as he evolved over the past forty-five years, from his departure from Harvard for Oxford in 1966 through the writing of his novels, the projects they worked on together, and the years of practice to the recent off-Broadway production of their play *Bill W. and Dr. Bob.* Stephen Bergman and Samuel Shem are the coauthors of "Resistance and Healing," in which they look back over the last thirty years.

The Birth of The House of God

DENIS NOBLE

It is so still that a match flame stands upright, invisible in the clear hot air. The green of the grass, the lime-white walls of our rented farmhouse, the orange stucco roof edging the August blue sky—it is all too perfect for this world.

SAMUEL SHEM, *THE HOUSE OF GOD*

CONCEPTION: FRANCE

It started in France. Yes, really. That's the title of the short introductory chapter. And those orange Roman roof tiles soaking up the hot sun to keep the old stone house cool, they are mine. They leaked badly then back in the 1970s. It cost me a small fortune to get someone up there to repair it all—a roof the size of a church roof!

Or perhaps it started in Morocco. As is usual in the matter of births, the causes are multiple. The parentage can even be confused. And then again, perhaps it started at the Balliol Graduate Centre at Holywell Manor in Oxford. The real Samuel Shem was a doctoral student at Balliol. But, of course, everyone who has read the book thinks it started at Beth Israel.

Well, they are all wrong. I know. I was there at its conception, not just at its birth. I see so many of the subtle influences that must have formed in Shem's mind. Perhaps he himself doesn't recognize all of them. So, here is my analysis of the conception.

My Périgord house is old and it is large. The main hearth is so huge that you can walk into it and burn logs the length of fence poles. But next door to it there is a much smaller house. Thirty years later, that one is also now part of my property, and each time I walk into it to get it ready for some guests, I ask myself a question. There are just two bedrooms and a living room. How on earth did it ever house five generations? For when Roy Basch was eyeing Berry's naked body, mopping up the artichoke juice and throwing the used leaves to the "glass-eyed gomer of a dog," Monsieur Perruchaud, a short but hefty man with the physique of the strong builder he was, lived in that small house with his wife, his mother, his ninety-five-year-old grandmother, two children, and two grandchildren! Oh, and the dog.

Well, I did once find an old bed in the loft, so perhaps the grandchildren slept up there. And part of the living room had been partitioned to allow for a third bedroom. Even so, where on earth did they all go? The point is, it didn't matter. In the old French country tradition, people lived on top of each other, and what was certain was that old granny, and even older great-granny, would never be turned over to a House of God (*maison dieu* in French is a poor people's hospice) except in the most extreme circumstances. Quite simply, they never became gomeres in that sense.

Of course, some did. Not everyone, even in the deep French countryside, has families to look after them. There is a *maison dieu* a few kilometers away in a beautiful cliff-side town just on the edge of the Dordogne. I am sure that Shem knew about that. It appears as the hospice referred to about four pages from the end of the book. I know the path he refers to only too well. It meanders up and down the steep cliff side on which the town is perched. I know the fabulous view that he describes so well. Deep inside the cliff, there is a huge sixth-century underground cathedral—the largest in Europe. Many of the gomers and gomeres of centuries ago are buried there. As Roy Basch is made to survey the demented people in the hospice, he has a totally changed view: "I love these gomers now." The return to France at the end of the book is an essential part of Shem's poetic vision.

So, what Shem knew when he wrote those lines was that many of the very old die quietly after years of care within their families. The same story could be repeated in most of the other families in the Dordogne villages. The contrast with the United States and the United Kingdom that must have formed in Shem's mind was surely part of the need to start the book with the scene in France. There are other reasons too. As I said, the parentage is not simple.

DECISION: MOROCCO AND OXFORD

Morocco? I see snake charmers, snail cooks, and Arabic storytellers in the huge old smoky square of Marrakesh, the last major town, pink buildings everywhere, before the journey out into the desert toward the Atlas Mountains.

Shem returned one day from those mountains in Morocco with a large Ali Baba earthenware pot that for many years accumulated green lichen where it was left in my garden. He had gone there on a break from doctoral thesis work on neurophysiology in my laboratory, working out how to make cockroaches lift their legs. The work had gotten to a critical stage, the stage where there was enough data to require analysis and modeling. Steve—for now that we are talking about the scientist, we had better give him his real name—had convinced me that we needed a computer. In those days, computers were something special. No question of cheap mass-produced desktops and laptops. These were serious big rack-mounted machines costing too much, and they arrived in a great stack of boxes. That stack was in the corridor waiting for Steve's return. Putting them together would make even the most complicated flat pack look like a piece of cake. The tangle of wires at the back resembled an old-fashioned telephone exchange.

I was at home—as head of the Graduate Centre, I lived at the beautiful sixteenth-century Oxford house called Holywell Manor—when a knock on the kitchen door announced the arrival of a hairy face, a bedraggled coat, and a bottle of wine. I now realize that the bottle of wine was a peace offering. Steve had already been to the lab and seen the pile of boxes. But he had also decided, somewhere on that Moroccan trip, that he was not—at least not yet—going to use that damn computer. Yet he had convinced me to beg, borrow, or steal the funds for that machine. He had every reason to think that I would be angry as he blurted out the truth over my kitchen table: "Denis, I'm not going to be a scientist; I am going to write!"

What he didn't know was that I had already sized up the situation. I have seen enough signs of students kicking against the straightjacket of an academic project. It was clear even before he went to Morocco that Steve was going to write. He came back from Morocco expecting to shock me. Instead I shocked him: "Well, Bergman, let's have a sherry!" We did, and we drank that bottle of wine. And somehow supper was rustled up in my kitchen from some lamb chops he had brought. It always was possible to rustle up supper. The team in my lab often came back late after an experiment to cook up curry, pasta, or whatever.

In an article written for the *Balliol College Record* two years ago, Steve gave his own version of this story. His words convey the story much better than mine:

It was one of those moments that change things for every other moment. Suddenly I saw him seeing me clearly, and I he clearly, saw what made him a brilliant scientist and authentic person and saw what made science wrong for me and—this is the remarkable part, for it had never happened to me before in my life—saw him seeing me and my life and where I had come from and where I would go, and *affirming* it. We started in on the sherry, and then—I had charged four lamb chops as well—on the dinner and on the wine.

And for some reason what flashed into my mind was how, just when you're looking hard for a camel auction you wind up at an olive harvest where you happen to come up against an awe-inspiring dancer and other stuff that changes your life for good. (Bergman 19)

So *The House of God had* to be born. Sometime. Though not quite yet. In fact, later, Steve did return to Oxford and completed his doctoral thesis. All those electrical traces were eventually analyzed and fitted to a set of equations. Did I say "fitted"? The computed lines went through the data somehow or other, and I was probably hoping to see the back of the project by then. My lab had moved on to other problems. Looking at the graphs with the eyes of a praying optimist, I told Steve that the fit was "jolly good." I must have told him though to check with Julian Jack. Julian was a serious mathematical neurophysiologist working just down the corridor—he could twist deconvolutions, Laplace transforms, and error functions through his hands and conjure up analytical equations by the ton—as indeed he did. We worked together on a massive mathematical treatise called *Electric Current Flow in Excitable Cells*. It is five hundred pages long, and it contains more equations than text!

Julian took one look at the data and the mathematically generated lines and went apoplectic. As he saw the lines veering this way and that, crazily avoiding the center of the points, he came straight to the blunt point. "Pretty bad" was his judgment. I think Julian would see a deviation, even by a whisker, from a mile off, and he just wasn't buying this one. It was more than a whisker. I don't know how that problem was eventually resolved, but Steve (or was it his mum?) told me once that his mother, after a visit back to the States, sent him off with a fierce look and a few choice words: "Remember, I want that degree!" He eventually got that doctorate.

One of the lessons I have learned in academic life is that it doesn't pay to force anyone along a line of inquiry that he really doesn't want to take. Moreover, I think it is the duty of a professor to detect the signs and allow the freedom that unusual talent requires. One member of my team at that time was not at all happy with the way I handled Steve's declaration. But, you know, the computer got used, and Steve kept coming back. What more could anyone want? Well, a book! But that is precisely what Steve delivered.

And what a book! He now tells me that the orgy scene was written while he was living with me at Holywell Manor. I might have guessed. Holywell, as its name suggests (the Holy Well), is a magical place. The ghosts are everywhere. I no longer live there, but we have left the ghosts of that orgy scene somewhere in the rafters to haunt Steve's and my successors.

THE MESSAGE

Years later, during one of those returns, we arranged for Steve to lecture to the student medical society. The day started with a special lunch in the old common room of the college. I had spoken with the chef and challenged him to produce a Périgord feast: a cassoulet of confit of duck, if I remember correctly. It was of course a reminder of where the book was conceived.

Later in the day, the medical school theater was packed for his lecture "How to Stay Human in Medicine." I guarantee that most had read *The House of God*. Even here in the United Kingdom, and most particularly at Steve's old college, it has become a must for medical students. Nor was it just the students who packed the theater. Hidden among them were many of the faculty who had crept in too. Steve gave a vintage performance. If there is one thing that he feels that is better than writing the book, it is surely lecturing on it to the young. As the Jesuits know only too well, forget the old: catch them young!

FALSE PROPHETS

And why should they be caught? Well, I'll tell you why. The problem that *The House of God* reveals is deep. It is not just the politics, the administration, the ethics, and the finance of health care. It is also a whole range of problems arising from the dominant twentieth-century philosophy of biology. That philosophy has a base formed fifty years ago when Watson and Crick did their Nobel Prize–winning work on the double helix. Very significantly, the base is called the central *dogma* of molecular biology, from which we get the notion that all information and causality flow from DNA through to proteins and then, by extension, through to all the other levels of organization. It never flows the other way.

Built onto the foundation of that dogma is the genes' eye view, popularized by *The Selfish Gene,* with the extraordinary insistence that genes "created us body and mind" (Dawkins 21). And in case anyone missed the message, one of Crick's last works, *The Astonishing Hypothesis,* contains the statement "You, your joys and your sorrows, your memories and your ambitions, your sense of personal identity and free will, are in fact no more than the behavior of a vast assembly of nerve cells and their associated molecules" (3).

These messages have been fed as gospel truths to generations of medical students. There are many malign consequences. They include the idea that for each disease there is a molecular explanation. Got cancer? Well, somewhere you were unlucky enough to have one of those "cancer genes." Sudden heart death? Sorry, you just had the wrong sodium channel mutation. Everything must have a particular molecular explanation. Medicine then becomes working out what those molecular problems are and fixing them. Of course, when it works, as with antibiotics killing bugs or insulin injections controlling diabetes, it's brilliant. But, taken as the dominant philosophy of medicine, it is dehumanizing. In *The House of God,* when someone dies in perfect electrolyte balance, the doctor can say with pride: "He went out The-House-of-God way!" (Shem 311).

Even worse than that: often enough it just doesn't work. Particularly as we age, diseases become multifactorial. As the ancient Chinese realized, you have to treat the whole person. When the Human Genome Project was launched a decade or two ago, the promise was that we would be able to read the book of life. Cures would then come tumbling out of that book. Well, the cures have been coming merely as a trickle, not an avalanche, and the book—well, it turns out to be a "machine language" database, not even a program, let alone a book.

The truth is that all the statements forming the twentieth-century philosophical foundation of biology are questionable or downright wrong (see Noble, "Claude Bernard," *Music of Life*).

A MORE HUMANE PHILOSOPHY?

First, the central dogma: no scientific hypothesis should ever be called a dogma since all scientific ideas are open to question and refutation.[1] Sure, so far as we know, protein sequences can never be back-translated into DNA sequences. In this limited sense, Crick's idea is almost certainly correct. But this limits the relevant information to the DNA sequences. That tells us which protein is coded for but not how much of that protein will be made. Yet this information, on relative gene expression levels, is what makes a heart cell different from, say, a bone cell or a pancreatic cell. Moreover, the epigenetic information that determines these expression levels does flow in the direction opposite to that implied by the dogma. It is cells and tissues that tell the genome how much of each protein to make. A heart cell divides into two heart cells, not two bone cells, because it marks the DNA with what are called epigenetic markers.

Second, gene determinism. *The Selfish Gene* has a lot to answer for. Even its author, Richard Dawkins, does not really believe what many people have interpreted it to mean. Genes do not "create us body and mind" (21). Dawkins even titles a chapter of one of his latest books "Genes Aren't Us" to acknowledge and emphasize that point (see Dawkins, *Devil's Chaplain*). The fact is that "selfish" is metaphorical (except perhaps in a limited mathematical sense having to do with kin selection and a form of altruism), and it can be seriously misleading. It is easy to demonstrate this fact. Simply take the central statements of *The Selfish Gene*, turn them upside down to state their opposites, and then ask, "Could any experiment possibly distinguish between the two?" The answer is a resounding no (Noble, *Music of Life*).

Third, *The Astonishing Hypothesis*. What is astonishing about this hypothesis is that it is almost impossible to make any sense out of it. Entities like the mind (the soul, if you will) simply do not exist at the molecular level. This is not a property peculiar to entities like the mind. It applies to all biological functions.

The rhythm of the heart, for example, is an integrative property of specialized cells in what is called the pacemaker region, the sinus node. There is no gene *for* cardiac rhythm. Instead there is a set of interactions between many gene products. The rhythm is a systems property, not a property of individual components (Noble, *Music of Life*).

Some readers of this essay will already have spotted where I am coming from. I believe that just as the twentieth century was the century of molecular biology, the twenty-first century will be that of systems biology. It is not easy to define what that means, though I have tried to do so in my own recent work (see Noble, "Claude Bernard," *Music of Life*). But it could be the antidote to what *The House of God* reveals as a problem in the philosophy of medicine and biology. The higher levels of the systems approach are, of course, the whole organism and the physical and social environments in which the organism functions. Inevitably, therefore, a science of medicine based on the systems approach must require its practitioners to return to treating the whole person. That is best done by respecting the person as a whole. There is no middle way.

If *The House of God* was a wake-up call highlighting the malign effects of a machinelike approach to treatment and medication, then a new biology is needed to answer that call. It will not replace the old, reductive mode. That will remain as one side of the coin, with integration on the other side. We return eventually to a concept dear to old traditional Chinese medicine: a duality of approach. Molecular biology is the yang of the duo. Systems form the yin. The union of yin and yang is the way forward.

The House of God contains a hint of this way forward, in the person of the Fat Man, the chief resident. Amidst the chaos, he holds to two basic redemptive ideals: authenticity—"Trash your illusions, and the world will beat a pathway to your door" (Shem 88)—and connection—"I make my patients feel like they're still part of life, part of some grand nutty scheme instead of alone with their diseases. . . . With me, they feel they're still part of the human race" (Shem 193). This is the hope in *The House of God*—a system that encourages doctors to use all the science at their disposal in a humane, healing way.

NOTES

1. Crick himself later recognized this mistake. In his autobiography he wrote:

I called this idea the central dogma, for two reasons, I suspect. I had already used the obvious word hypothesis in the sequence hypothesis, and in addition I wanted to suggest that this new assumption was more central and more powerful. . . . As it turned out, the use of the word dogma caused almost more trouble than it was worth. . . . Many years later Jacques Monod pointed out to me that I did not appear to understand the correct use of the word dogma, which is a belief that cannot be doubted. I did apprehend this in a vague sort of way but since I thought that all religious beliefs were without foundation, I used the word the way I myself thought about it, not as most of the world does, and simply applied it to a grand hypothesis that, however plausible, had little direct experimental support. (*What Mad Pursuit* 182)

WORKS CITED

Bergman, Stephen J. "The Computer and the Belly Dancer: On Becoming a Writer at Balliol." *Balliol College Record* (2005): 18–22.

Crick, Francis. *The Astonishing Hypothesis: The Scientific Search for the Soul.* London: Simon and Schuster, 1994.

———. "Central Dogma of Molecular Biology." *Nature* 227 (1970): 561–63.

———. *What Mad Pursuit: A Personal View of Scientific Discovery.* London: Penguin Books, 1990.

Dawkins, Richard. *A Devil's Chaplain.* London: Weidenfeld and Nicolson, 2003.

———. *The Selfish Gene.* Oxford: Oxford University Press, 1976.

Jack, James, Julian Bennett, Denis Noble, and Richard W. Tsien. *Electric Current Flow in Excitable Cells.* Oxford: Oxford University Press, 1975.

Noble, Denis. "Claude Bernard, the First Systems Biologist, and the Future of Physiology." *Experimental Physiology* 93 (2008): 16–26.

———. *The Music of Life.* Oxford: Oxford University Press, 2006.

Residency Education in Historical Perspective

Houses of God before Shem:
Boston City and the Thorndike at Bellevue

GERALD WEISSMANN

Ye worthy, honored, philanthropic few,
The muse shall weave her brightest wreaths for you.
Who in Humanity's bland cause unite,
Nor heed the shaft by interest aimed or spite;
Like the great Pattern of Benevolence,
Hygea's blessing to the poor dispense;
And though opposed by folly's servile brood,
ENJOY THE LUXURY OF DOING GOOD.

C. CAUSTIC, *TERRIBLE TRACTORATION*

Doctors come of professional age in their house staff years: habits are rehearsed, skills honed, friendships set for life. Life as a resident at a teaching hospital combines aspects of an army recruit's basic training with a lawyer's clerkship in chambers. I spent those wonder years on the busy public wards of Bellevue Hospital in the late 1950s, where one soon learned that the drill book we were following had been written in Boston.

In his first year as chief of medicine of the III and IV medical divisions at Bellevue, Lewis Thomas asked me to be his chief resident. He told me not only that I'd be on call every night and day, with alternate weekends off, but also that he wanted his chief resident to have a laboratory next to his, adjacent to the open public ward in the A&B building. (I had been a postdoctoral fellow of Severo Ochoa and was pleased by that proposal.) Thomas also considered the chief residency he was offering as the first step to a career in academic medicine. "This place is going to be like the Thorndike and Boston City!" he told me. I was still deciding whether to follow my father into practice or move on to an academic career in science. When Dr. Thomas told me what academic salaries were like in the late 1950s, my impertinent younger self quoted in dismay: "What is science but the absence of prejudice in the presence of money?" "Henry James," said Lewis Thomas, "from *The Golden Bowl*, chapter 1." He went on, "All right then, you won't earn very much but you'll have a lot of fun in the lab and time to read." My dad never did have much time. I have remained at NYU–Bellevue ever since. While life on the wards at Bellevue has often recapitulated the catch-22 antics of *The House of God*, at our best we adhered to another model, that of Boston City and the Thorndike.

After the First World War, the Harvard Medical Unit at Boston City Hospital and its associated Thorndike lab had reformed the way medicine was taught and practiced in municipal teaching hospitals. Medical training programs country-wide soon followed Boston's dictum that laboratory and clinical experience were indispensable to each other, and both necessary for the training of young physicians. One could bring science from the bedside to the lab bench and back again—and also serve the medically needy. The Boston City/Thorndike model was a caring and curious doctor who could enjoy the luxury of doing good. The house staff memoirs of the Harvard Medical Unit at Boston City Hospital at its zenith in the 1930s are a tribute to doctors and patients alike (Finland and Castle 336). They are also the story of medicine before Medicare and Medicaid and penicillin.

In the thirties, Harvard was responsible for the second and the fourth of the five medical services at Boston City Hospital; the others were directed by Boston and Tufts universities. Of these, perhaps the most prestigious was the fourth, which was housed in the Peabody building, a structure connected to the Thorndike labs by "bridges" on which patients were housed in times of overcrowding. Boston City Hospital was an institution both charitable and commercial. On one hand, the poor—"those incapacitated from taking care of themselves," in the words of its 1860 prospectus (qtd. in Rosenberg 136)—were treated at little or no cost to themselves; on the other hand, they paid their fee in the coin of medical instruction. Their illnesses became "cases," the raw material that medical students, house officers, and attending physicians turned into the textbook of clinical medicine (Rosenberg). The best and the brightest of Harvard shuttled between those labs and the wards: the history of the Harvard Medical Unit at Boston City Hospital proudly announces that of the seventy-one young physicians who trained there between 1936 and 1940, fifty-two became professors of medicine, while six went on to medical school deanships (Finland and Castle xxvi).

PUPS AND SENIORS

Interns at the Boston City Hospital in the 1930s signed up for an apprentice-ship in internal medicine that would last eighteen months. The interns were expected to work their way up a steep ladder in six rotations of three months each. Beginning as a "pup," who was mainly expected to do the scut work, the novice rotated through a period of outpatient service, followed by another three months of tending to the infectious diseases ward. Then came the reward for those first nine months of dog's work: "the privilege of giving the orders instead of receiving them" (Thomas 38). The intern became, in turn, a senior physician (the senior who looked after the pup), an assistant house physician, and, finally, the house physician. Nowadays, the "house" would be called the chief resident. There were no residents at Boston City in the modern sense of the term; after a year and a half of internship, one simply went into practice or was called into the academy.

Nowadays critics of "paternalistic, hieratic" medicine complain that the patients were warehoused thirty or more to each open ward to serve the role of human guinea pigs. They tell us that the poor were piled bed upon bed like so much industrial inventory for the convenience of doctors, that charity cases provided the fodder of medical teaching (Rosenberg 339). But the memoirs of Finland, Castle, and their colleagues at Boston City Hospital paint an entirely different picture. On the contrary, they show that the charity patients were the center of a busy hospital life, in which families, friends, clergy, doctors, nurses, medical students, interns, and custodians formed a community. In the days of the Great Depression, patients in the City Hospital found themselves in a precinct that was cleaner, warmer, and more caring by far than any slum in Boston. The records also show that in 1937, as in 1860, doctors and patients were parties to a barter agreement—care was given in exchange for teaching—a largely amicable contract that was unbreached for over a century before it was annulled by the HMOs: "The hospital was part of an institutional world [in which] physicians were paid in prestige and clinical access; trustees in deference and the opportunity for spiritual accomplishment; nurses and patients were compensated with creature comforts: food, heat and a place to sleep. Patients offered deference and their bodies as teaching material. Few dollars changed hands, but the system worked in its limited way for those who participated in it" (Rosenberg 229).

Those directly involved had more visceral responses. Here are some diary entries of William L. Peltz, an intern on the Peabody Service of Boston City Hospital in the winter of 1938:

· To bed at 2:30 A.M. after working 18½ hrs, one hour's sleep and now a new patient to be admitted at 3:30 A.M. Age 55 diabetes with gastritis, says the supervisor's office. We'll see!
· Maria de Sista, aged eighteen with her TB on Peabody 2. She helped out with housework in the home of a woman who had TB. That was 4 years ago, and the woman has since died at Rutland [a TB sanitarium]. But Mary didn't know that at the time. A swell kid! Wanted to get married next April and now has advanced TB on the right. Came in spitting up blood. She began three months

ago when she might have had a halfway decent chance, but some "friend" said not to worry, it was nothing, so she didn't bother going to the doctor.

· Anastasia O'Neil, who looks sixty-three but says she's seventy-four, who must weigh 250 pounds but says she's 150, who was sent in by her doctor with a note saying she has severe diabetes but who hasn't required insulin yet. "Sure an' they don't know what diabetes is in the old country; an' when yer sick the old folks know where to go out in the fields an' pick a big bunch o' herbs. Gee the hospital is a swell place; an' the City Hospital is as good as any place you can get."

· Diabetes! Anyway it is now 5:30. Now for two hours sleep—hopefully! (I am not up for alcoholics.) (297)

It's hard to remember now, but before the Second World War, medical services of the great teaching hospitals provided mainly custodial, rather than remedial, care: food, heat, and a place to get well. The doctors might relieve pain and suffering, but they had few real remedies in hand. They could give arsenic for syphilis, insulin for diabetes, raw liver for pernicious anemia, and antisera for pneumonia. But by and large, as one of them recalled, "Whether you survived or not depended on the natural history of the disease. . . . And yet, everyone, all the professionals, were frantically busy, trying to cope, doing one thing after another, all day and all night" (Thomas 40). Busiest of all were the interns.

Bill Peltz, who was to become a professor of psychiatry at Penn, described the intern's work as "typing blood, doing urinalyses and examining stools, giving transfusions, taking EKGs, typing pneumococci, pronouncing people dead and signing death certificates" (297). The interns were also expected to work in the emergency room and the outpatient department from which they rushed back to the wards to start IVs, perform catheterizations, measure basal metabolism, do spinal taps, place tubes in various orifices, "and more and more." Once past the pup stage, the interns admitted sick people at the rate of four or five per night, obtained their patients' social and medical histories, performed physical examinations, did all but the most difficult laboratory examinations, and, after mulling over all other possibilities, committed themselves to the single most likely diagnosis and plan of treatment. Then they waited. Over the next few hours, days, or weeks, they watched—but rarely influenced—the disease until the patient got better or worse; they were again required to keep detailed records of what happened. It was called "keeping," or later, "buffing," the chart. Interns were also expected to comfort their patients, to make accurate prognoses, and, when all had come to naught, to beg permission from the patient's nearest relative for an autopsy. In the course of these efforts they were expected to work every day and every other night, to ignore weekends—and to remain unmarried.

In return, the interns received room and board and medical training that would last a lifetime. Franz J. Ingelfinger, who was Lewis Thomas's senior and later the best medical editor of his day, remembered looking up at the stars—or as much as could be seen between the Peabody building on one side and the house officer's building on the other—and imploring the deities that he might do a good job: "It was an emotional and heady walk between those buildings" (Finland and Castle 313). Thomas himself had fond recollections of the time: "I am remembering the internship through a haze of time, cluttered by all sorts of memories of other jobs, but I haven't got it wrong nor am I romanticizing the experience. It was, simply, the best of times" (36).

Many of those who worked on the Peabody wards and at the Thorndike Memorial Laboratory agreed. "My experience on the Harvard Medical services was the most intense of my life," claimed a future professor of medicine in Seattle, Bud Evans (Finland and Castle 353).

Nowadays, when brokers' apprentices or bimbos in Washington are called "interns," we tend to forget that the title "intern" derives from the Parisian teaching hospitals of the middle of the nineteenth century, which rewarded their best and brightest students with an *internat*. The losers in the intellectual lottery were awarded an *externat* (Weissmann, *Democracy* 36). Looking back at the memoirs of the Boston City days, I'm amused by the recent externalization of the internship. I remain convinced that the title of "intern" should be reserved for those who tend the sick *inside* a teaching hospital, those who live and work and sleep there, those who have enlisted to be on call, as one used to say.

Internship, then as now, had its pleasures as well as its trials. Five months into his internship, Thomas celebrated in doggerel a gift that Mr. Maloof, a grateful fifty-three-year-old "Assyrian crock," gave to the doctors who had taken care of him. The gift was a curiously hammered brass pot that went to Peltz, who as house physician had first call on gifts. Cary Peters (assistant house) and Ingelfinger (the senior), who also appear in the poem, were further down the line of command. Thomas slipped into an office on Peabody 3 and typed an "Ode to a 90-Year Old Assyrian Pot," which concluded:

And didst thou hope. Oh Burnished Pot
That such a fate should be thy lot?
That thou wouldst be so doubly blest:
To leave Maloof and be the guest
Of someone else?
Of William Peltz?
Oh happy Pot! Oh lucky toss!
Maloof came in while Peltz was boss!

For if he'd chose at home to tarry
Thou mights have gone to Peters, Cary!
And if he'd longer chose to linger
Thou mights have gone to Ingelfinger!
But no! Thou goest to no one else
But Dr. William Learned Peltz! (337)

On Christmas morning of 1937, Thomas crossed over to the house officer's building to post a note on his senior's door; it had been written in the dead of night on Fourth Medical:

Of Christmas joys I am the Bringer;
I bring good news to Ingelfinger
Though many turned in bed and cried
Nobody died! nobody died! (337)

A photograph has survived of these men sitting before the house officers' building in the early fall sunshine of 1937 (Lawrence 38–39). Thomas is the senior of the group and is seated with Alexander Burgess and Bud Evans, his pup. They are three good-looking, neatly scrubbed young American doctors in crisp whites sporting white buck shoes. Thomas has a percussion hammer poking from the breast pocket of his starched tunic. The three men look at us across the years as if they knew, as Evans recalled, that the times had the attributes of the end of an era. It was certainly the end of a period of do-it-yourself activity in internal medicine.

For instance, cross-matching blood at night and giving blood in kits sterilized by the house staff must have ceased shortly after this. Typing pneumococci and giving antipneumococcal serum during the night also adds glamour in retrospect that was removed when it became possible to prescribe sulfonamide and go to bed (Finland and Castle 353).

And yet that do-it-yourself experience became indelible. Richard Ebert, a future chairman of medicine at Minnesota, expressed it for them all: "I developed a self-reliance and a knowledge of my clinical competence.... The experience tested our abilities to withstand stress. The internship was a kind of indoor Outward Bound" (Finland and Castle 304). Those days come to life in Bill Peltz's casebook of 1937–38 on the Peabody Service. The sound is that of the Popular Front:

· Mannie Sample, the great brown colored girl in the Sun Room 1 whose toes I pinch and who has a laugh I like to hear.
· Catherine Healy who has diabetes and pyelitis and whom we have had in here

twice now, damn near dead each time. Once with a tidal drainage going and the second time coming in insulin shock.

- Bessie Johnson, the little colored girl with pneumonia, who wrote me afterward as I hoped she would. I remember the night she was crying because she heard she was going to a convalescent home and how she called me over.

- Ventura Bocafuscia, the swell old Italian on the Peabody 1 bridge with his bigeminal pulse. He would teach me Italian each day. It was always a pleasure to make rounds past his bed because he was so cheerful. And his rhythm straightened out after quinidine.

- And Henry Coffin who ... when he was operated on they found a huge ulcer too big to do anything for and he died a few days later.

- Going around on the Peabody 1 and 2 the last night and saying goodbye to all the patients and nurses and the ward help. Saying goodbye to Dr. [Soma] Weiss and the futile effort to express your sadness and regret. (298)

THE LONG WHITE COATS

The house officers were under the spell of Soma Weiss and the other Young Turks of the Harvard Unit, who "moved back and forth between the Peabody building and their laboratories in the Thorndike ... in long white coats. They came at ten in the morning to make the formal rounds, walked the bedsides for two or three hours with the interns and medical students, and they came back at odd hours throughout the afternoon and often until late in the evening to see patients with serious problems in whom they were especially interested" (Thomas 38).

Chief of that glittering Harvard Medical Unit was George C. Minot. It did not escape house-staff notice that one could be a teacher, a clinician, and a scientist all at once. Minot and his predecessor, Francis Weld Peabody, who had put the Thorndike together from scratch, combined each of those roles. Scions of distinguished Boston families, they were also regarded by their house officers as avatars of the Brahmin physician. Interns on the Peabody Service of the Boston City Hospital had each been given a copy of Peabody's *Doctor and Patient;* many of them knew key passages of the book by heart.

Sporting a brisk introduction by Hans Zinsser, Peabody's *Doctor and Patient* provided generations of Harvard physicians with the rhetoric of clinical idealism—much in the way that William Osler's *Aequanimitas* summed up the strictures of an earlier era (Weissmann, "Against *Aequanimitas*" 211). Peabody's book revealed the mind of a doctor who could link the art and science of medicine—and who could write about both. Peabody's dictum "The treatment of a disease may be entirely impersonal; the care of the patient must be completely personal" became a watchword for a generation of house officers (877).

Even more widely quoted was the last sentence of Peabody's essay "The Care of the Patient": "The good physician knows his patients through and through, and his knowledge is bought dearly. Time, sympathy and understanding must be lavishly dispensed, but the reward is to be found in that personal bond which forms the greatest satisfaction of the practice of medicine. One of the essential qualities of the clinician is interest in humanity, for the secret of the care of the patient is in caring for the patient" (882).

At the time, Peabody was one of only two full-time professors of medicine at the Harvard Medical School (Aub and Hapgood 279). Publication of his essay as the lead article in the *Journal of the American Medical Association* in 1927 and the simultaneous publication of his scientific work on pernicious anemia constitute a milestone in the history of academic medicine in America. I remember reading the following passage early one morning in the chief resident's bunk at Bellevue Hospital in 1959, when I was wondering whether a career in full-time medicine would help or hinder my ability to care for patients:

> The most common criticism made at present by older practitioners is that young graduates have been taught a great deal about the mechanism of disease, but very little about the practice of medicine or, to put it more bluntly, they are too "scientific" and do not know how to take care of patients. . . . When a patient enters a hospital, one of the first things that commonly happens to him is that he loses his personal identity. He is generally referred to, not as Henry Jones, but as "that case of mitral stenosis in the second bed on the left." There are plenty of reasons why this is so, and the point is, in itself, relatively unimportant; but the struggle is that it leads, more or less directly, to the patient being treated as a case of mitral stenosis, and not as a sick man. (82)

When Peabody died, his shoes were filled by George Minot, and his path was followed by the young men he had brought to the Thorndike. *Primum inter pares* among these was the Hungarian-born Soma Weiss (1899–1942). Weiss's brief meteoric career assumed some of the aura of that of Xavier Bichat, the founder of modern tissue pathology in the Napoleonic era (Aub and Hapgood 279). Weiss grew up in a Hungarian mountain town, the son of a successful civil engineer. In response to the anti-Semitic turbulence of Budapest after World War I, Weiss arrived in New York in 1920 and is said to have applied at the same time, and with success, for American citizenship and admission to Cornell University Medical College, then located directly across the street from Bellevue Hospital. After internship at Bellevue, Weiss was attracted to the Thorndike by Peabody, where Peabody's Young Turks were busy "running a laboratory, teaching on the wards, and providing research training for young doctors" (Thomas 38).

Weiss was an enthusiastic teacher, an unflagging clinical researcher, and an effective administrator. Among his various accomplishments were the first description of how patients fainted in the "carotid sinus syndrome" (which he demonstrated by projecting the shadow of the quartz filament of an old electro-cardiograph on the front wall), the introduction of intravenous sodium amytal (first used to relieve the severe contractions of tetanus), and measurement of the circulation time at the bedside (by means of histamine or vital dyes). With George P. Robb, he first showed that paroxysmal nocturnal dyspnea (waking up short of breath in the middle of the night) was caused by overload of the left ventricle. These days his name remains in our literature as half of an eponym for the Mallory-Weiss syndrome: a rupture of the esophagus because of sus-tained vomiting, as after one has had too much alcohol (Beecher and Altschule 303–7). The house staff remembered him best as *the* man to call on when on long winter nights there was a question to be answered or a patient to be seen. He was "always about."

Weiss showed the same unflagging energy when he became chief of the second and fourth services. William Bean, a future professor at Iowa and a faithful scribe of medicine, remembers that Weiss's bedside demonstrations were models of clarity and often a virtuoso's tour de force: "His Hungarian accent, which lent charm to his almost dangerously attractive personality quite unconsciously intensified at certain times and almost vanished at others" (Finland and Castle 267). Alexander Langmuir, the future chief epidemiologist of the CDC, recalled that the thirty-four-year-old Weiss was constantly on the wards: "He was never dull. Then in a flash he was off, always running with his white coat tails flying" (Finland and Castle 252). He was deeply concerned about each patient and never let his interns forget the slightest detail of clinical management. He insisted that the interns not be diverted by the countless medical fascinations of the Boston medical scene, even the excellent libraries, until they had worked up all their cases completely.

Said Weiss: "You will never again have a chance to see human disease as it unfolds each hour day and night, under your eyes on the wards. You can hear distinguished lectures and read journals the rest of your life." It was a restate-ment, for Boston, of Osler's famous dictum that he who observes patients without studying books is like one at sea without a chart. But he who studies books without observing patients is like one who has never been to sea at all (Finland and Castle 252, 267). The rounds began early in the morning and often ended late at night, when Weiss and his wife (Elizabeth Jones Weiss) entertained interns and fellows at home: "The Weiss's home was a happy holiday haven for homesick fellows," recalled Bean (Finland and Castle 268), while Paul Kunkel, a future Yale professor, recalled that one of the fondest memories he had of

Weiss was the intimate Sunday evening buffets at home where he, his charming wife, and their children presided. Invariably they had faculty from the liberal arts, who would keep conversation flowing at a lively pace (Finland and Castle 323). Scores of Thorndike alumni remember best those Wednesday evening rounds, when the house staff of all the Boston City Hospital medical services, Boston University, and Tufts as well as Harvard would present Soma Weiss with the toughest and most puzzling clinical cases. Kunkel remembers that "Soma carried a small black notebook that he peeked at occasionally after examining the patient and while still listening to the presentation, and I do not recall he was ever in error" (Finland and Castle 322). Often, after having come up with the correct diagnosis, Weiss would end his remarks with "I've seen it again and again!" (Finland and Castle 140).

At age forty, Weiss was appointed the Hersey Professor of the Theory and Practice of Physic and physician-in-chief at the Brigham Hospital, Harvard's most prestigious academic chair. Sadly, Soma Weiss's time at Brigham was brief, because in December 1941 he was stricken by a severe headache that he correctly diagnosed himself as a subarachnoid hemorrhage. One month later he was dead. The house officers of the day always regarded Weiss as the most engaged teacher they had ever met: those nights on the wards, the warmth of the Sunday buffets, the keen questions to the point, Weiss was one of those who made it the best of times for a young intern.

When I was chief resident at Bellevue in the fifties, not very much had changed: Minot and Peabody, Weiss, and Peltz would have felt at home. The training was still a bit like boot camp, and the indigent patients of our big city hospital were still warehoused on open wards. Antibiotics, diuretics, and cortisone had, of course, become available, and the interns—the best and brightest of Bellevue—were able to do a good bit more for their patients, but young diabetics continued to be admitted with recurrent bouts of pyelitis, little "colored" girls came in with pneumonia, and grown men died of huge ulcers after futile operations. An intern's life at Bellevue in the fifties was as it was at Boston City in the thirties: the constant busywork; those hours on open, overcrowded, and underheated winter wards; those nights spent looking at blood and urine; the intense drive to be of use. Those who worked on Lewis Thomas's service at Bellevue Hospital wouldn't have gotten it wrong either. For us it was also, simply, the best of times. But Thomas would also have been the first to argue the point that nostalgia is no substitute for quick and certain knowledge. By the eighties, Thomas knew that there was no going back: "Medicine is no longer the laying on of hands, it is more like the reading of signals from machines. . . . There is no changing this, no going back; nor, when you think about it, is there really any reason for wanting to go back. If I am in a bed in a modern hospital, worrying about the cost of that bed as well, I want to get out as fast as possible, whole if possible" (38).

NOTES

This essay is adapted from one originally published in *Pharos* 68.4 (2005): 14–20, and published here by courtesy of the Alpha Omega Alpha Honor Medical Society.

WORKS CITED

Aub, Joseph C., and Ruth K. Hapgood. *Pioneer in Modern Medicine: David Linn Edsall of Harvard.* Boston: Harvard Medical Alumni Association, 1970.

Beecher, Henry K., and Mark D. Altschule. *Medicine at Harvard: The First 300 Years.* Dartmouth, NH: New England Universities Press, 1977.

Caustic, Christopher. *Terrible Tractoration! A Poetical Petition Against Galvanizing Trumpery....* 1804. Quoted in Oliver Wendall Holmes, "Homeopathy and Its Kindred Delusions," 1842 in *Medical Essays* (Boston: Riverside Press, 1892 edition).

Finland, Maxwell, and William B. Castle, eds. *The Harvard Medical Unit at the Boston City Hospital.* Vol. 2. Boston: Countway Library of Medicine HMS, 1983.

Lawrence, H. S. "Presentation of the George M. Kober Medal to Lewis Thomas." *Transactions of the Association of American Physicians* 96 (1983): cxviii–cxxxiv.

Peabody, Francis W. "The Care of the Patient." *Journal of the American Medical Association* 88 (1927): 877–82.

———. *Doctor and Patient.* New York: Macmillan, 1931.

Rosenberg, Charles. *The Care of Strangers: The Rise of America's Hospital System.* New York: Basic Books, 1987.

Thomas, Lewis. *The Youngest Science: Notes of a Medicine-Watcher.* New York: Viking, 1983.

Weissmann, Gerald. "Against *Aequanimitas.*" *The Woods Hole Cantata.* New York: Dodd, Mead, 1985. 211.

Weissmann, Gerald. *Democracy and DNA.* New York: Knopf, 1995.

Residency Education since The House of God

KENNETH M. LUDMERER

Immediately on publication, Samuel Shem's brilliant novel *The House of God* struck a nerve among American physicians. However, medical opinion about the book was far from unanimous. As the author himself reported, younger doctors loved the book, while older physicians pilloried him for having written it. Younger doctors claimed the book spoke the truth about the brutalities and inhumanities of residency training; senior physicians considered the novel a mockery of the serious, dignified process of transforming a callow medical student into a mature physician.

In this essay, I shall attempt to demonstrate two points: first, that Shem's account of residency training in the United States accurately portrayed the conditions of residency it satirized, and, second, that the underlying conditions that led to fatigue, burnout, and cynicism among residents working in the House of God have not substantively changed in the three decades since the appearance of the novel, even as medical educators have made efforts to transform residency into a kinder, gentler experience. Graduate medical education by its very nature demands that a delicate balance be struck between education and service. The essence of the house officers' dilemma in the House of God—and today—is that this balance has been heavily tilted toward service. This balance must be redressed, and the educational component of residency training reaffirmed, if we are finally to make residency training a more humane and educationally effective experience.

GRADUATE MEDICAL EDUCATION BEFORE AND AT THE HOUSE OF GOD

To understand the experience of the house officers at the House of God, it is necessary to understand the history and traditions of residency training in the United States. Before World War I, medical education in America focused almost exclusively on "undergraduate" medical education—the years of study at medical school leading to the MD. At a time when the great majority of medical school graduates entered general practice, the four years of medical school were considered an adequate preparation for the practice of medicine. Abraham Flexner's heralded 1910 report on medical education did not even mention internship or other hospital training for medical graduates, reflecting the prevailing orthodoxy that the four years of medical school provided sufficient preparation for general practice.

By World War I, however, medical knowledge, techniques, and practices had grown enormously. There was too much to teach, even in a four-year course. Accordingly, a period of hospital education following graduation—the internship— became standard for every physician (Ludmerer, *Time to Heal* 79–90). Medical education in the early twentieth century also faced the challenge of meeting the needs of individuals who desired to practice a clinical specialty (such as ophthalmology, internal medicine, or surgery) or to pursue a career in medical research. To this end, a several-year hospital experience following internship—the residency—became the accepted vehicle (Ludmerer, *Time to Heal* 79–90). This period of formal medical education after medical school came to be known as graduate medical education (GME).

Two educational principles lay at the heart of GME. First, the defining characteristic of GME was the assumption of responsibility by house officers for patient management. It was axiomatic in medicine that an individual was not a mature physician until he or she had learned to assume full responsibility for the care of patients. To acquire this capacity, interns and residents evaluated patients for themselves, made their own decisions about diagnosis and therapy, and performed their own procedures and treatments. Responsibility was graded—that is, the more senior the house officer, the more responsibility was allowed. House officers were supervised by and accountable to attending physicians. Nevertheless, they were allowed considerable clinical independence. To seasoned educators and clinicians, this was the best way for learners to be transformed into mature physicians and to develop the capacity for the independent practice of medicine. (By "independent practice of medicine," medical educators meant the ability of a physician to work safely without supervision, not without the collaboration of other health care professionals.)

Second, medical educators emphasized repeatedly that the caseload of house officers should not be too heavy. It was far better for the intellectual growth of residents, they argued, for house officers to study fewer patients in depth rather than more patients superficially. No less an authority than Abraham Flexner spoke to this point. "Men become educated by steeping themselves thoroughly in a few subjects, not by nibbling at many," he wrote in 1925 (*Comparative Study* 148). Scientific method was best taught through the "intensive and thorough study of relatively few patients" (270). This educational principle was honored at the better teaching programs. For instance, in 1939 interns at teaching hospitals carried an average load of nine patients at a time, compared with an average load of twenty-five patients at a time among interns at community hospitals (Graduate Medical Education 10, 76–77, 255). The lower number of patients at teaching hospitals allowed house officers there more time to read, attend conferences and rounds, engage in clinical research, and monitor their patients carefully.

Few experiences evoked such an extraordinary range of emotions as residency. The innumerable stresses were real: hard work, long hours, sleepless nights, the sense of vulnerability to unpredictable forces like nursing shortages and summertime heat waves, and the pressures of being responsible for every aspect of patient care. Yet these stresses were countered by the camaraderie among the resident staff, the feeling of being part of a family, the deep satisfaction of making a difference in people's health and lives, and the exhilaration of being aware that one's medical competence was growing perceptibly almost daily. Thus, with hindsight, most doctors have viewed the experience nostalgically. This helps explain why older physicians reacted so negatively to *The House of God*. Far removed from their own residencies, and much better rested, they had forgotten the harshness of residency training and now remembered only its more enjoyable features.

Nevertheless, from the very beginning, a fundamental dilemma plagued GME. Was the training education or service? Were house officers students or hospital employees? As with other dualisms, the answer was both. It was impossible to separate the educational from the service components of GME because the fundamental pedagogic principle of internship and residency called for house officers to develop independence by assuming responsibility for their patients' total care. However, the amount of service actually required for learning was far less than that which hospitals and medical faculties typically extracted from house officers. A tradition of the economic exploitation of house officers began, as hospitals from the start insisted that trainees perform an extraordinary range and amount of ancillary responsibilities. It was the degrading and abusive aspects of residency that younger doctors, fresh from the experience, still remembered when they read *The House of God*.

Even in the 1920s and 1930s, house officers were regularly exploited as a source of inexpensive labor. The greatest deviation from educational ideals occurred at community hospitals not affiliated with medical schools. At some of these hospitals, interns were considered subordinate to nurses and permitted only to take routine histories and administer intravenous medications. Didactic rounds, teaching conferences, and other educational activities were very few. However, even at the best programs, the amount of routine work could be overwhelming. At major teaching hospitals, house officers were deluged with innumerable duties—performing blood counts and urinalyses, transporting patients to X-ray or physical therapy, drawing blood samples, and starting intravenous lines—that hardly needed to be performed by a physician. Complaints of too little teaching and too much scut work were commonplace (Ludmerer, *Time to Heal* 82–83).

Such problems were highlighted in 1940 in the *Report of the Commission on Graduate Medical Education,* the first report on graduate medical education in the United States. This report took dead aim at the economic exploitation of interns and residents. To improve the educational value of graduate medical education, first and foremost hospitals "must work out plans to relieve the intern [and resident] from many routine procedures which he is now performing but which have relatively little educational value" (Graduate Medical Education 59). After the noneducational responsibilities are removed, the next step to improve graduate medical education is "expanding its educational content" (60). According to the report, hospitals should hire salaried physicians rather than interns and residents if they could not make adequate educational opportunities available to house officers.

Nevertheless, such pleadings went unheeded. As hospitals expanded the size of their residency programs after World War II, the delicate balance between education and service remained heavily tilted toward service. The continuing subjugation of education to service led to many additional calls for residency programs to take their educational responsibilities more seriously. For instance, in the 1960s the Millis report, sponsored by the American Medical Association, and the Coggeshall report, sponsored by the Association of American Medical Colleges, challenged residency programs to lessen the workloads placed on house officers. However, residency programs failed to do so. Indeed, workloads remained so heavy that in the 1970s house officers at many programs attempted to unionize (Ludmerer, *Time to Heal* 243–49).

Thus, notwithstanding the many literary licenses taken in the book, the experiences of Roy Basch and his colleagues in *The House of God* represented an accurate portrayal of residency training in the United States in the 1970s. At training programs everywhere, house officers worked under conditions of extreme stress. Overwork, sleep deprivation, constant fatigue, cynicism, the sense of powerlessness and isolation, the feeling of being vulnerable to impersonal forces, and the perverse view that the patient was the enemy were commonplace among interns and residents. One published study of sleep deprivation among medical interns in 1971 observed that not only impaired performance but also negative mood swings and transient psychopathology could result (Friedman, Bigger, and Kornfeld). Of course, at the House of God and elsewhere, the experiences of residency were made bearable by the unusually close and collegial relationships house officers had with each other. And there were innumerable rewards to residency training, most notably, the recognition that one was becoming competent as a physician.

But at the House of God and in American medical education writ large, residency training was far more frantic and difficult than it had to be. The reason for this was the longstanding tradition in GME of subordinating education to service.

GRADUATE MEDICAL EDUCATION FROM *THE HOUSE OF GOD* THROUGH THE PRESENT

During the past three decades, GME in the United States has continued to evolve. One conspicuous trend is that the academic emphasis originally found in residency programs has markedly declined. As noted before, an initial goal of residency was that of training the next generation of clinical investigators. Accordingly, research represented an important component of the residency experience. After World War II, as the amount of clinical knowledge grew and as clinical research became more sophisticated, residency programs began to focus more and more on clinical learning alone. In this context it is noteworthy that research was not even mentioned in *The House of God*. Over the past three decades this trend has continued. Often today, residents have the opportunity to participate in research electives. However, this experience is insufficient to prepare them to be mature, independent clinical investigators during the present molecular era of clinical research. Aspiring physician-scientists who need the heavy dose of basic science training necessary to conduct contemporary clinical research need to acquire that experience elsewhere.

Second, the sense house officers once had, and that was so apparent in *The House of God*, of belonging to a metaphorical family has significantly lessened. In part this is because the number of residents in many programs grew so large. For instance, in 2007 there were nearly 150 residents in internal medicine alone at Barnes-Jewish Hospital (the teaching hospital of the Washington University in St. Louis School of Medicine), compared to 22 in 1970. In addition, the decline of community has resulted from the disappearance of faculty from the wards. Faculty today remain readily available to provide help. However, after rounds they are typically off, with full schedules of private patients to see or important experiments to conduct. Most professors today have little time to get to know house officers on a personal level or to serve as bedside role models. Accordingly, few house officers speak any longer of heroes in the profession or describe their training in terms of the individuals under whom they work. Even fewer speak of any spiritual uplift they might derive from the experience of being a member of the resident staff.

Third, over the past three decades GME has remained primarily an inpatient experience, even though technological developments have been allowing many more conditions to be managed effectively and safely on an outpatient basis.

With the exception of programs in family practice and pediatrics, outpatient education remains rarely emphasized, in part because the financing of GME is linked to inpatient care, and in part because of the traditional disdain of medical faculty toward outpatient instruction.

Lastly, the pace of house staff life has grown ever more frenetic, as patients have become sicker, technologies more sophisticated, and nights on call busier. In the 1960s intensive care units were introduced, as were new life-sustaining technologies like ventilators and dialysis machines. By the 1980s these were all commonplace. Everywhere in the hospital the pace became more hectic, as organ transplantation became more routine, cancer chemotherapy rapidly advanced, and the diagnosis of end-stage disease of any kind often carried the possibility of another treatment rather than resignation to death. Mastery became required of a host of sophisticated technologies: Swan-Ganz catheters, Holter monitors, electrical cardioverters, pacemakers, new classes of antibiotics, and intravenous pharmacologic agents to raise or drop a person's blood pressure in seconds. Reinforcing these conditions was a common cultural characteristic of residency programs; that is, the idea that house officers had to demonstrate that they had the "right stuff" to be physicians by handling any problem and any amount of work without calling for help.

To add to the pressures of house staff training, in the 1980s residents began admitting many more patients than before. The residency had been created in an era when relatively stable patients lingered in the hospital for long periods, and a cardinal educational tenet of GME was that house officers should study patients in depth. In 1984, the introduction of prospective payment for hospitals greatly increased the patient load of house officers. As a result of prospective payment, residents immediately began admitting two or three times the number of patients per admitting day, and the average length of stay at teaching hospitals dramatically fell. For house officers in all fields, this meant busier days and nights, less time to read and sleep, and greater stress, tension, and fatigue (Ludmerer, *Time to Heal* 357–62). The overwork and exhaustion did perverse things to the caring individuals who entered medicine to serve, as acting out among residents was common. So were stress-related depression, emotional impairment, and alcohol and substance abuse (see Aach, Girard, et al.; Resident Services Committee; Smith, Denny, and Witzke).

As during earlier eras in GME, the plight of residents was made more difficult by the many extraneous duties they had to perform, such as drawing bloods and inserting intravenous lines. The tradition of taking economic advantage of house officers continued unabated. In the 1970s, most teaching hospitals began to provide house officers greater assistance with some of these tasks. More phlebotomists and technicians were hired, and nurses were given greater authority to perform certain procedures. However, these steps provided residents little relief from scut work for telephone calls, scheduling chores, and dictations, and time spent charting increased even as the time consumed by manual procedures decreased (Katz and Schroeder; Lurie, Rank, et al.).

The dilemmas of residency training were thrust into the public spotlight in 1984, following the death of eighteen-year-old Libby Zion at the New York Hospital. Ms. Zion had presented to the hospital with the seemingly minor complaints of fever and an earache; eight hours later she was dead. Her family alleged that her death was the result of overwork and undersupervision of the medical house officers who cared for her, and the district attorney of Manhattan convened a grand jury to investigate those charges.

Despite years of review by various medical and legal groups, the cause of Libby Zion's death was never determined. The house officers in the main acted appropriately. They were not fatigued, and they were in communication by telephone with Ms. Zion's private physician. The grand jury refused to indict the doctors on criminal charges, and the state medical board did not revoke their licenses. Nevertheless, the grand jury did indict the system of residency training in the United States, and the case became a cause célèbre for limiting the work hours and increasing the supervision of house officers (Spritz, Farber, Robins).

The grand jury report led to the creation of a special commission headed by Bertrand N. Bell, professor of medicine at the Albert Einstein College of Medicine, which, after nineteen months of deliberation, issued a series of recommendations on the working hours and supervision of residents. These recommendations were incorporated into the New York State Health Code in July 1989. New York was the only state to pass such legislation, but similar regulations were voluntarily enacted by most of the residency review committees that governed residency training in the various specialties. Specifics varied from one field to another, but in general the new regulations called for a restriction of the resident workweek to eighty hours averaged over four weeks, the mandatory provision of one day off per week, limitations on the lengths of shifts in the emergency room, and the requirement of greater direct supervision by attending physicians. Only the residency review committees in surgery and the surgical subspecialties did not pass such regulations.

Unfortunately, the new rules were widely disregarded. One study of graduate medical education throughout the nation in the 1998–99 training year found that nearly half of postgraduate year 1 residents and one-third of postgraduate year 2 residents reported working more than eighty hours per week (Baldwin, Daugherty, et al.). Ironically, compliance with work-hour regulations was especially bad in New York State, which had mandated work-hour restrictions by law. In 1998, 37 percent of all residents in the state reported working more than eighty-five hours per week, and 20 percent, more than ninety-five hours per week (DeBuono and Osten). A major reason for the disregard of the requirements was the continued reliance of hospitals on house officers for routine tasks. Bertrand Bell himself pointed out that New York's new regulations on hours were "being widely flouted" because interns and residents were still "too frequently exploited as cheap labor" (A15).

The issue of residency work hours resurfaced in 1999 when the National Labor Relations Board overturned a twenty-three-year precedent by ruling that residents at private institutions could unionize and enter into collective bargaining. The release of the Institute of Medicine's widely discussed report *To Err Is Human* intensified the debate. With mounting concern about medical error, patient safety, and the deleterious effects of long work hours on residents' physical and emotional health, a political tidal wave to restrict hours erupted. In June 2002 the Accreditation Council for Graduate Medical Education (ACGME), the organization that accredits residency education programs, announced new regulations, effective July 1, 2003, limiting the number of hours worked by residents to eighty hours of work per week, averaged over a four-week period. (Starting July 1, 2004, programs could petition the ACGME for an additional eight hours per week, provided they could offer an educational justification for those hours.) The regulations also mandated that residents be on call in the hospital no more than every third night; that continuous duty be limited to twenty-four hours, with an added period of up to six hours for continuity and transfer of care and didactic activities; that residents have at least ten hours off between work periods; and that house officers receive at least one day off out of every seven. Had the ACGME not acted, it is likely that even more restrictive regulations would have been imposed by Congress (Steinbrook).

The new ACGME regulations triggered an enormous and ongoing controversy. Defenders of the ACGME regulations have justifiably pointed to the many problems associated with sleep deprivation, excessive stress, and the lack of a balanced life (Glines; Mukherjee; Ofri; Drazen; Skeff, Ezeji-Okoye, et al.). Critics have worried about the loss of continuity of care, a possible rise in medical mistakes because of poor information transfer during the "handoff," and the loss of opportunity for residents to gain as much medical and surgical experience as in the past. Particularly galling to many critics has been the rigidity and inflexibility of the new regulations, which require a resident to stop work by *precisely* a certain time. Such a requirement, they argue, shifts the gaze of the resident away from the patient to the clock, promoting the development of a shift mentality. Scheduling has become a time-devouring nightmare for chief residents and program directors, and the attendance of house officers at grand rounds and other educational conferences has dwindled. Sleep while one is on call counts toward the eighty hours, while moonlighting outside the institution does not. To further confound the situation, the decision to make the workweek eighty hours rather than some other amount of time was purely arbitrary, and good data about the effects of various work schedules on resident health, clinical performance, and educational and patient outcomes are scarce (Barone and Ivy, Charap, Darves, Fischer, Schroeder).

From a historical and educational perspective, the great problem with the new ACGME regulations is that the regulations have not resolved, and have probably worsened, the problem they were intended to correct: house staff stress. Residents now have more time off, but nights on call are still arduous and long, and the amount of work is even greater since there are now more patients to admit each on-call day. Moreover, despite an ACGME requirement that hospitals add more support staff, it is not apparent that they have done so adequately to relieve the resident workload. Consequently, as always, this work falls to the house staff. One study found residents in all disciplines devoting as much as 35 percent of their time to activities of either marginal or no educational value (Boex and Leahy). The new rules do not guarantee adequate amenities while residents are on call, a faculty that knows and cares about the house staff, stimulating conferences and rounds, the ready availability of advisors and mentors, a fair policy regarding parental leave, the immediate accessibility of help, and a strong sense of camaraderie. The new rules certainly do not guarantee residents enough time to evaluate and study their patients thoroughly. The limitation of working hours, in short, says nothing about the larger issue of working conditions. The good intentions of the ACGME aside, the regulations perpetuate and probably aggravate the tradition of subordinating education to service in GME.

Given the trajectory of GME from the beginning, this situation should hardly be a surprise. There has never been a time when GME in the United States has realized its own educational ideals. The chief problem has been the ongoing subordination of the educational aspects of residency to institutional service needs. This was clearly demonstrated in *The House of God;* it remains true today. The lesson to be learned is that GME must be judged by the total experience, not by the hours of work alone. Medical educators need to pay attention to what house officers do with their hours, not merely how many hours they put in. It is crucial that professional leaders understand this point if GME is to be made better.

RESTORING THE BALANCE

Can GME be transformed into the invigorating experience it was meant to be? From a historical and educational perspective, the answer is yes, but four tasks need to be accomplished to allow this to happen.

First, and most important, medical educators once again need to provide trainees the opportunity for detailed study of patients. This can occur only if learners receive sufficient time—time for meaningful clinical encounters, time for critical thinking, and time for study and reflection. Since prospective payment was introduced two decades ago in an effort to control hospital costs, this cardinal educational principle has been ignored. House officers have been functioning as evaluation machines, admitting many more patients a night than before, all to keep the service covered and hospital throughput at a high level, but at a significant cost to their education (Ludmerer, *Time to Heal* 357–62).

It is imperative that this fundamental educational principle once again be honored. There must be a major reduction in the number of patients residents are expected to work up per admitting day. For this reduction to occur, teaching hospitals will need to reengineer themselves so that they become less dependent on house officers for the provision of patient care, which will require the greater use of hospitalists, fellows, and other physicians, as well as nurse-practitioners, physician assistants, and other health care workers. Faculty will have to revisit what they do. For instance, faculty might have to do some of their own evaluations and write-ups, and attending physicians might have to run a service without house officers. The cardiovascular service at the Mayo Clinic has already reported a successful experiment with this approach. They created a new service consisting of a team of cardiovascular attending physicians, cardiovascular fellows, nurse-practitioners, physician assistants, and registered nurse liaisons—but no internal medicine residents. Educational and clinical outcomes were eminently satisfactory, as was the satisfaction with the experiment among house officers, attending cardiologists, and patients (Nishimura, Linderbaum, et al.).

Second, residents must be relieved from chores that have minimal educational value and that can be done equally well by nonphysicians. This requires the provision of more nurses, technicians, clerks, transporters, IV teams, blood drawers, and other supportive staff. It also requires more assistance with all the scheduling issues and discharge planning that have become such a conspicuous part of contemporary hospital medicine. Such changes have already been occurring at many hospitals, but these organizational changes need to be accelerated and made permanent.

Third, residency programs need to focus on maintaining and improving the quality of educational opportunities they offer. Greater attention must be given to the array of conferences, seminars, rounds, and other formal and informal educational activities important to GME. Even more attention must be given to encouraging residents to attend these activities. It would be refreshing to see the ACGME encouraging residents to attend educational events with the same vigor it now requires house officers to leave the hospital when their shifts are over.

Efforts also need to be made to bring faculty back to the teaching units—not only for direct teaching and supervision but for the establishment of personal relationships. Of course, the same present-day pressures on faculty to increase "clinical productivity" that have taken faculty out of the lives of medical students have had similar consequences for residents. However, medical faculties have ample opportunity to bring clinical teachers back to teaching, provided they are willing to place a higher priority on the educational mission than they were in the past (Ludmerer, "Learner-Centered Medical Education"). Indeed, many have already started to do so via a greater willingness to promote clinician-educators, as well as through the adaptation of "academies of medical educators," mission-based budgeting, and other strategies to raise or identify funds to pay teachers for teaching.

Fourth, training programs need to work hard at changing the culture of GME so that stress is decreased and the experience is more responsive to the emotional needs of trainees. This means much more than providing house officers with amenities like parking, meals, and comfortable on-call quarters. It also means providing such opportunities as split residencies for house officers with young children and ready access to help. It is essential that department chairs, training program directors, and faculty truly care about the welfare of their residents, and that the residents know that they care. Faculty must work hard to counter the traditional mind-set that a resident who is not around all the time is not a good physician. In the past, residents were taught that the best way to learn medicine was to spend more time on the floors. Faculty and trainees must be taught that the best way to learn medicine is to invest time wisely. In a related vein, program directors need to eliminate the cowboy mentality of the resident and make certain that house officers can ask for help without fear of recrimination.

A common denominator to these suggestions for reforming residency training is that they are expensive. No hospital, however willing, can carry out the types of proposals made here unless third-party payments are sufficient to make that allowable. Unfortunately, in the current market-driven health care environment, third-party payments to hospitals are more restrictive, which forces institutions everywhere to retrench. In addition, hospitals are operating under an enormous regulatory burden that adds profoundly to their expenses. Funds that easily could be spent for more nurses, technicians, and computer systems are siphoned off to satisfy regulatory requirements, many of which are far removed from patient care and education. Teaching hospitals are in the paradoxical position of being criticized by the public for working their house officers too hard, yet they are often without sufficient resources to lessen the workload of residents appreciably. Given the centrality of GME to the quality of medical care available in America, it would seem foolhardy for the public not to support GME adequately, particularly given the huge amount of money the nation already spends on health care.

Teaching hospitals must also be prepared to use internal sources to provide additional funds for the support of GME. Can they achieve further operational efficiencies without affecting the quality of care and the service expected by patients and their families? Can they cap or cut back on the size of the rapidly expanding administrative staffs found at so many of them? Have they adequately protected existing educational funds by making certain that federal GME payments (which go directly to teaching hospitals, not to training programs) are fully distributed to the intended recipients? Perhaps most important, given that compensation guidelines reflect the values and mold the behavior of organizations, can the boards of teaching hospitals create compensation plans that reward senior hospital executives for the quality of medical work the institution does rather than for merely coming in below budget? I recognize that margins are necessary to fulfill mission, but bonuses and other financial incentives based solely on margins might tempt some administrators to skimp on mission. In short, teaching hospitals must be able to demonstrate that they have the institutional competency to use resources wisely.

GME in the United States has much to be proud of. On balance, for more than a century it has served the public well. Nevertheless, its history is one of a persistent failure to live up to its own ideals. With the astonishing complexity of modern medicine and the extraordinary demands on today's physicians, the need to address the deficiencies of GME has become urgent. The key to doing so is to establish, at last, the primacy of education over service.

WORKS CITED

Aach, R. D., D. E. Girard, et al. "Alcohol and Other Substance Abuse and Impairment among Physicians in Residency Training." *Annals of Internal Medicine* 116 (1992): 245–54.

Baldwin, D. C. Jr., S. R. Daugherty, et al. "A National Survey of Residents' Self-Reported Work Hours: Thinking beyond Specialty." *Academic Medicine* 78 (2003): 1154–63.

Barone, J. E., and M. E. Ivy. "Resident Work Hours: The Five Stages of Grief." *Academic Medicine* 79 (2004): 379–80.

Bell, B. M. "Greenhorns in White." *Wall Street Journal* 9 Feb. 1995: A15.

Boex, J. R., and P. J. Leahy. "Understanding Residents' Work: Moving beyond Counting Hours to Assessing Educational Value." *Academic Medicine* 78 (2003): 939–44.

Charap, M. "Reducing Resident Work Hours: Unproven Assumptions and Unforeseen Outcomes." *Annals of Internal Medicine* 140 (2004): 814–15.

Citizens Commission on Graduate Medical Education. *The Graduate Education of Physicians.* Chicago: American Medical Association, 1966.

Coggeshall, L. T. *Planning for Medical Progress through Education.* Evanston, IL: Association of American Medical Colleges, 1966.

Darves, B. "Work Hour Rules Rile Educators—and Residents." *ACP Observer* Oct. 2003: 1, 8–9.

DeBuono, B., and W. Osten. "The Medical Resident Workload: The Case of New York State." *Journal of the American Medical Association* 280 (1998): 1882–83.

Drazen, J. M. "Awake and Informed." *New England Journal of Medicine* 351 (2004): 1884.

Farber, M. A. "Who Killed Libby Zion?" *Vanity Fair* Dec. 1988: 190–95.

Fischer, J. E. "Continuity of Care: A Casualty of the 80-Hour Work Week." *Academic Medicine* 79 (2004): 381–83.

Flexner, Abraham. *Medical Education: A Comparative Study.* New York: Macmillan, 1925.

———. *Medical Education in the United States and Canada.* New York: Carnegie Foundation for the Advancement of Teaching, 1910.

Friedman, R. C., J. T. Bigger, and D. S. Kornfeld. "The Intern and Sleep Loss." *New England Journal of Medicine* 285 (1971): 201–3.

Glines, M. E. "The Effect of Work Hour Regulations on Personal Development during Residency." *Annals of Internal Medicine* 140 (2004): 818–19.

Graduate Medical Education. *Report of the Commission on Graduate Medical Education.* Chicago: University of Chicago Press, 1940.

Katz, M. H., and S. Schroeder. "The Sounds of the Hospital: Paging Patterns in Three Teaching Hospitals." *New England Journal of Medicine* 319 (1988): 1585–89.

Kohn, L. T., J. M. Corrigan, and M. S. Donaldson, eds. *To Err Is Human: Building a Safer Health System.* Washington, D.C.: National Academy Press, 2000.

Ludmerer, Kenneth M. "Learner-Centered Medical Education." *New England Journal of Medicine* 351 (2004): 1163–64.

———. *Time to Heal: American Medical Education from the Turn of the Century to the Era of Managed Care.* New York: Oxford University Press, 1999.

Lurie, N., B. Rank, C. Parenti, et al. "How Do House Officers Spend Their Nights? A Time Study of Internal Medicine House Staff on Call." *New England Journal of Medicine* 320 (1989): 1673–77.

Mukherjee, S. "A Precarious Exchange." *New England Journal of Medicine* 351 (2004): 1822–24.

Nishimura, R. A., J. A. Linderbaum, et al. "A Nonresident Cardiovascular Inpatient Service Improves Residents' Experiences in an Academic Medical Center: A New Model to Meet the Challenges of the New Millenium." *Academic Medicine* 79 (2004): 426–31.

Ofri, D. "Residency Regulations—Resisting Our Reflexes." *New England Journal of Medicine* 351 (2004): 1824–26.

Resident Services Committee, Association of Program Directors in Internal Medicine. "Stress and Impairment during Residency Training: Strategies for Reduction, Identification, and Management." *Annals of Internal Medicine* 109 (1988): 154–61.

Robins, N. *The Girl Who Died Twice: The Libby Zion Case and the Hidden Hazards of Hospitals.* New York: Delacorte Press, 1995.

Schroeder, S. A. "How Many Hours Is Enough? An Old Profession Meets a New Generation." *Annals of Internal Medicine* 140 (2004): 838–39.

Skeff, K. M., S. Ezeji-Okoye, et al. "Benefits of Resident Work Hours Regulations." *Annals of Internal Medicine* 140 (2004): 816–17.

Smith, J. W., W. F. Denny, and D. B. Witzke. "Emotional Impairment in Internal Medicine House Staff." *Journal of the American Medical Association* 255 (1986): 1155–58.

Spritz, N. "Oversight of Physicians? Conduct by State Licensing Agencies: Lessons from New York's Libby Zion Case." *Annals of Internal Medicine* 115 (1991): 219–22.

Steinbrook, R. "The Debate over Residents' Work Hours." *New England Journal of Medicine* 347 (2002): 1296–302.

From The House of God *to the House of Siemens:*
Bedside Skills Thirty Years Later

SARAH LAPEY, JUDY MCCARTER, AND ABRAHAM VERGHESE

The House of God begins the summer after Roy Basch has survived his internship; he is in France, recuperating and relearning how to live with his girlfriend, Berry. Even though he is on holiday, however, his medical training does not take a vacation: he notices the waiter in the restaurant has a "senile tremor" (Shem 4). Similarly, when walking past a medical facility, he has an involuntary reaction: "My skin prickles, the little hairs on the back of my neck rise, my teeth set on edge. And there, sure enough, I see them. I recognize the signs. I make diagnoses" (7). This kind of observational skill—being able to spot diseases at a glance—speaks of a sophistication that comes from many hours of bedside training. Still, such talent does not spare him from dehumanizing his patients or feeling dehumanized himself. Roy bemoans the outcome of his internship year, during which he "had been hurt, bad. For before the House of God, I had loved old people. Now they were no longer old people, they were gomers, and I did not, I could not, love them any more" (5).

The narrator does, however, celebrate the lessons learned, and the most enduring insights arise from his resident, the Fat Man, whose "zany laughter and . . . caring . . . had gotten [him] through the year" (5). The Fat Man is a fountain of physical diagnosis observations. As Roy's first resident and a fresh survivor of his own internship, he is also a type of bard, embodying vision, perspective, and practicality, combined with humor and cynicism. He speaks the truth. He recognizes the senselessness underlying the patient management led by the private attendings in which a patient admitted with depression and headaches will be ordered "the complete gastrointestinal workup, consisting of barium enema, upper GI series, small bowel follow-through, sigmoidoscopy, and liver scan" (32). This, he says, is "doing medicine the House of God way" (33), and while linked to financial gains for the private physicians, as well as new hospital buildings like the "Wing of Zock" (33), it results in mindless, illogical work for the house staff.

Thirty years after *The House of God,* our hospitals are transformed: the charts have been replaced by computerized medical records; sophisticated imaging that might have been the product of the Fat Man's vivid imagination are now the norm. Such diagnostic modalities, along with intricate genetic and molecular level assays, have allowed us to be fairly precise about what ails the patient, and what *will* one day ail the patient. But this has come with an increased feeling among patients that medicine has become impersonal, that it revolves around technology and procedures.

More importantly for physicians, the ease and availability of such testing have resulted in an atrophy of bedside medicine skills and a corresponding lack of faith both in their own simple senses and in the time-honored skills that have allowed physicians to say with certainty that there is fluid around a lung, that the mitral valve is stenosed, or that the liver is enlarged. We would make the argument that if medicine and science continue to progress, so to speak, in this fashion, one could postulate that a patient claiming to be missing a finger would not be credible until he or she is armed with an X-ray or a bone scan—trained senses simply do not suffice in this time of technology. In contrast, what is re- markable is that in the fictional world of *The House of God*, bedside skills were very refined, as in this scene: "In hushed silence we stood in the middle of the dimly lit Rose Room. All was still, spectral, the four Roses horizontal, at peace, barely dimpling their swaddling sheets. It was all very nice, until the smell hit" (231). The stench was such that the three interns and three medical students, "yelping and retching, handkerchiefs to their mouths," proceeded to flee from the room. Only the Fat Man remained. He argued, "You can learn a lot from that aroma. With luck, in three months you'll be able to stand in the middle of that room and give the four diagnoses as the different bowel odors smack your olfactory lobes. Why, just today there was a steatorrheac malabsorption, a bowel carcinoma, a superior mesenteric insufficiency giving rise to bowel ischemia and diarrhea, and last? . . . yes! Little packets of gas slipping past a long-standing fecal impaction" (231).

Not only do images of clinical examination and physical diagnosis—by the bedside, in the hospital corridors, and overflowing into everyday life—abound in *The House of God,* but the novel also foreshadows the demise of the skills referred to earlier because of today's significantly greater reliance on technology. Other factors in the decline include a training process that is much busier than it was in the Fat Man's or Roy's days; increased turnover of patients because of shortened stays; a grave threat to the continuity of care due to limits on house officers' hours of duty; and finally, a reimbursement system that rewards proce- dures (because they are easier to quantify) and refuses to similarly honor bedside clinical skills. A further threat to physical examination skills is the aging and impending retirement of a generation of teachers—the Fat Man being of that generation—who relied on bedside skills at least to some degree. In the scene we quoted about noxious odors, the Fat Man demonstrates perhaps one of the most significant attributes of skilled examiners, namely, faith in the process, a willingness to examine and trust what the basic senses convey about their patients, and finally an understanding of life and illness that enables them to empathize with the situation and the patient.

There are further demonstrations of such faith: as the ward team marches down the corridors, Fats points out physical findings on the patients they pass, such as the O and Q signs (230), in which the degree of mouth droop and protrusion of the tongue serves as a prognosticator for recovery. When a patient immobilized in restraints following a long, sleepless night is found at the nursing station Fats explains the concept of "Sundowning" (47). His twist on the usual approach to fall precautions is to provide his patients with a "Los Angeles Rams football helmet" (37). We can see the influence of Fats's keen observation skills on Roy's prose: he describes the hospital as a "huge urine-colored building" (16) and its corridors as "bile-colored" (26). He notes a "horrific purple birthmark" (16) on the face of the chief of medicine and registers the "magnificently hairy forearms" (26) of a ward's nurse. Potts's young patient in the hallway receives the nickname "the Yellow Man," reflecting that he is "yellow from liver disease" (42).

In stark contrast to the Fat Man is the resident Jo. She is described as the "most ruthless and competitive resident" (86), and her credo is "the more you do in medicine, the better care you give" (86). Exceptionally driven, she rounds earlier than Fats so that she can see all the patients and investigate their medical problems meticulously. Despite her intense motivation to deliver excellent medical care, Jo lacks clinical maturity so that she is unable to appreciate big-picture issues and is also awkward and blind in her interpersonal interactions. This results in her overreliance on technology.

"'Start ordering the tests,' said Jo . . . 'We're really going to work this up. Completely. No one's going to be able to say that we do sloppy work'" (88). While Fats recognizes the importance of seeking simple and practical interventions for patients to improve their quality of life, such as providing new eyeglasses for Anna O, an elderly patient with dementia, Jo struggles to grasp the issues of most relevance to this fragile patient. As a result, Jo orchestrates for Anna O a complete dementia workup, including a battery of radiographic studies and a lumbar puncture, all of which trigger a sad downhill decline for the patient. Roy bears witness:

Given the stress of the dementia workup, every organ system crumpled: in a domino progression, the injection of radioactive dye for her brain scan shut down her kidneys, and the dye study of her kidneys overloaded her heart, and the medication for her heart made her vomit, which altered her electrolyte balance in a life-threatening way, which increased her dementia and shut down her bowel, which made her eligible for the bowel run, the cleanout for which dehydrated her and really shut down her tormented kidneys, which led to infection, the need for dialysis, and big-time complications of these big-time diseases . . . she became very sick. (90)

When Roy discusses Jo's "go-all-out" approach to medical care with the Fat Man, Fats is able to recognize the way in which Jo's difficulty connecting with people, stemming from her own life of imbalance and depression, prevents her from making a difference in the medical care she provides: she's a "terrific medical text lacking in common sense . . . [and] a klutz when it comes to practical medicine and human contact" (91).

The Fat Man is a humanist and displays genuine empathy and appreciation for human connections with both patients and colleagues. It's clear that his interns appreciate this on their first day, when Fats tells them, "I know how scared you new 'terns' are today" (28). This contrasts with the approach of the chief resident, nicknamed the Fish, of whom Roy says: "Shifty, slimy, he oozed. Too cheerful. Not in touch with our dread" (16).

So it comes as a shock to find that, despite the Fat Man's obvious skill at clinical observation, Fats concludes that these skills are neither needed nor particularly valued when the coin of the realm is doing the "workup" on each patient, securing the test results, and discharging patients.

Indeed, the grueling and inhumane training process seems to have taken the Fat Man's initial idealism and twisted it into a realism that keeps him sane. For all his skills, he decides to adopt a practice of avoiding physical contact with patients during house staff rounds. On the first day of wards, the Fat Man surprises the team with his declaration: "In internal medicine, there is virtually no need to see patients. Almost all patients are better off unseen. . . . These fingers do not touch bodies unless they have to. . . . I've seen enough bodies, and especially bodies of gomers, to last me the rest of my life" (27–28). Fats's system for work rounds, a shift from the classic bedside rounds accompanied by a patient chart rack, is termed the "card-flip" (30) in many hospitals. Sadly, today, this practice of "rounding" on patients while sitting in a conference room has become very common; the most important person in this exercise—the patient—is not present. "Card-flip" is an ironic term in *The House of God,* but it has come to be seen as anything but ironic.

Of course, there is danger in overemphasizing bedside skills, as illustrated in a scene where Dr. Donowitz, one of the "higher-up Slurpers" (16), brings the team to the bedside during a new patient presentation with a promise: "Let me show you a bedside test for amyloid" (37). He then "reached down and twisted the skin on the patient's forearm. Nothing happened. Puzzled, he said something about 'sometimes you have to do it a bit harder' and took hold of the skin, wadded it up, and gave it a tremendous twist. The patient gave a yelp, leaped up off the mattress, and began to cry with pain. Donowitz looked down and found that he'd ripped a big chunk of flesh from the guy's arm. Blood was squirting from the wound. Donowitz turned pale and didn't know what to do. Embarrassed . . . he ran out of the room" (37). The Fat Man, in contrast, remains grounded and calm. He "put a gauze compression bandage on the wound" (37). He then highlights the physical finding that "uremic skin is brittle" (37) and warns of the potential for infection. Days later, cultures from the iatrogenic wound showed "the Fat Man was right. Colorful and esoteric bacteria grew out of the wound, including one species that was native only to the rectum of the domestic duck" (38).

While the Fat Man may at times be casual and aloof, described as lounging with his "feet up, reading, ostensibly into the world of stocks and bonds and commodities" (39), he is also forever prepared and attuned to the needs of the interns and patients. "Like a king who knows his kingdom as well as he knows his own body. . . . He seemed to have a sense for any problem on the ward, instructing us, forewarning us" (39). When a newly admitted patient, Leo, unexpectedly codes in the midst of conversation and laughter, interns Roy and Potts freeze. Fats, on the other hand, springs into action, performing a one-person code team while Potts and Roy stand paralyzed in the periphery. "He thumped Leo, breathed Leo, closed-chest-cardiac-massaged Leo, IV'd Leo, and organized with a cool virtuosity Leo's cardiac arrest and Leo's return from the world of the dead" (40). The Fat Man similarly bounds to the assistance of Roy during an LP and acts as a coach, demonstrating his expertise in procedures: "With a smooth and effortless Sam Snead stroke, [he] sliced through the fat and popped into the subarachnoid space" (59). More importantly, Fats is also attuned to the emotional state of his interns, anticipating their potential for self-destructive feelings of failure as they make mistakes. In contrast to the chief resident, who overemphasizes shortcomings when intern Potts fails to give steroids to a patient in fulminant liver failure, Fats comforts Potts by saying, "I know how shitty you feel. There's no feeling like it in the world. If you don't feel it at least once, Potts, you'll never be a good doc. It's all right" (49).

That the Fat Man has been a good teacher is evident in a scene toward the end of Roy's internship, when Roy's clinical maturity and commonsense skills in bedside diagnosis are contrasted with those of a medical student, "789, or Sev," as they go to see a new transfer from orthopedics, Olive O. The medical student, recognized to be an "intellectual prodigy with few social skills" (332), had already done a comprehensive chart review of the patient's history, spoken with the collaborating orthopedics team, and reported seeing the patient and obtaining an EKG.

At the bedside with Roy, however, the patient they see doesn't appear to be the one described by the record, a patient who is known to have an amputated leg. The medical student then realizes that he saw the wrong patient and had overlooked the mismatch. He says, "I looked, I just didn't see the other leg, that's all. My cognitive set was for one leg, not for two" (333). As Roy reviews the physical examination findings with Sev, they encounter a rare unexplained presence of "two protrusions from the vicinity of her chest-belly. . . . Sprouting from her abdomen, below her low-slung flat breasts, were two humps" (333). Roy's approach to this perplexing finding is a fine illustration of his practical approach to a mysterious clinical finding. While the medical student says, "I've never heard of humps in humans. What's in 'em?" Roy determinedly responds, "Don't know, but, by God, we're gonna find out," as he begins to examine them (333).

A powerful sense of disillusionment with medicine as a clinical and curative art is revealed by the end of the book; Roy takes his black physician bag, so much a symbol of the practice of medicine, swings it over his head, and throws it into the wind. "Like a discus, round and round and round it went, gathering momentum, until with a scream of bitterness and joy, [he] launched it up and up into the fresh summer breeze and watched the glittering chrome instruments fall out in a rainbow and smash on the pavement below" (375–76). This scene is a striking contrast to the beginning of the internship. At that time, on the first day, the intern Potts had been described as "dressed in crisp white, pockets bulging with instruments" (27). Similarly, Roy, in his first attempts to see his inpatients, had described himself thus: "In a doctor costume, I took my black bag and entered their rooms" (32).

Clearly, by the end of the novel, Roy shares the disappointment of his fellow intern, Potts; his previous hopes for medicine are now "just a dream. . . . Not the kind of medicine I'm learning here" (214). Unlike Potts, who was overcome with despair and disenchantment with medicine and ended up taking his life, Roy is able to recognize a new meaning in medicine, which he learns from Fats. He no longer views the goal of medicine as seeking a cure but rather recognizes that medicine is about "being with people" (340) and experiencing a connection.

As Fats sees it, "The cure is the disease. The main source of illness in this world is the doctor's own illness: his compulsion to try to cure and his fraudulent belief that he can" (193). As Roy sees Fats modeling caring and compassion with his clinic patients, he has an epiphany: "Here is what medicine could be: human to human" (193).

Roy discovers with his own patients that they "didn't give a damn about their diseases or 'cures'; what they wanted was what anyone wanted: the hand in their hand, the sense that their doctor could care" (194).

Sir William Osler was clairvoyant in his observation that "to study the phenomenon of disease without books is to sail an uncharted sea, while to study books without patients is not to go to sea at all" (qtd. in Silverman, Murray, and Bryan xxvi). In *The House of God*, the primary importance of the connection between humans is recognized, and not only within the doctor-patient relationship, but also in the relationships of the health care staff, their families, and surrounding communities. Roy's girlfriend, Berry, recognizes that "the caring in your bunch of guys sustained you" (379). The intern Chuck also noted, "How can we care for patients if'n nobody cares for us?" (364).

In reflecting on *The House of God* thirty years later, we recognize the desensitization and potential disillusionment that can occur to a physician under the huge pressures of today's medical system; it is as true now as it was then.

While physicians may always share an enthusiasm for the "performance" side of medicine involving advances in technology and procedures, this cannot come at the cost of connection with the patient. Going to the bedside will always illuminate the concerns most pressing to the patient.

A recent experience on rounds with medical students serves as a good example of the importance of the skilled bedside exam for its own sake: while examining an elderly, largely silent patient with a respiratory problem, the attending began to percuss the patient's chest, mapping out the extent of a fluid collection around the chest. At this point, the patient broke out in a huge smile and said, "My doctor used to do that when I was a kid. Boy, he sure knew what he was doing."

At least from the patient's perspective, the laying on of hands, the use of one's senses as an adjunct to the many tests he had been subjected to, seemed to indicate both attentiveness and competence. Thirty years after *The House of God*, the secret to the care of the patient (to paraphrase Francis Weld Peabody[1]) is just as it was then, and that is in *caring* for the patient; nothing conveys that with quite the same certainty and ease as the artful elicitation of the history, the careful and skilled exam—putting one's hands on the humps (which ideally should lead to the judicious ordering of tests). Roy's observation is timeless and instructive for students today: what matters is "the hand in their hand, the sense that their doctor could care" (194).

NOTES

1. "For the secret of the care of the patient is in caring for the patient" (qtd. in Oglesby 817–18).

WORKS CITED

Oglesby, Paul. *The Caring Physician: The Life of Dr. Francis Weld Peabody.* Boston: Countway Library of Medicine, 1991.

Shem, Samuel. *The House of God.* New York: Dell, 2003.

Silverman, Mark E., T. Jock Murray, and Charles S. Bryan, eds. *The Quotable Osler.* Philadelphia: American College of Physicians, 2003.

The Godless Kingdom:
Medical Education in France, 1973–2008

MARC ZAFFRAN (MARTIN WINCKLER)

Like many physicians, I am the son of a doctor. My father the doctor was a great storyteller. I became a listener without giving it too much thought or effort. When I was a child in the 1960s, he loved to tell me stories about his own childhood, and narrating his medical training was something he enjoyed even more—probably because he enjoyed being a doctor and was grateful that the God he believed in had let him become one. His family was poor, he was an orphan (his father had died a soldier on the battlefield in 1915), and it wasn't too easy for a young Jewish man to become a doctor in early twentieth-century French-ruled Algeria. I had great admiration for my father. He was the kind of man bums went straight to in the street, and I never saw him turn any of them away. His hand was reaching for his pocket before they said their first word. He was a gentle, angry man. Gentle with people who were in pain. Angry with those who used their status for power. He felt a doctor's duty is to care. He infected me with these feelings.

Being that specific doctor's son was a unique experience. I was probably no more than ten when he started telling me about his days in Algiers's med school in the late 1930s. He not only taught me to listen to stories; he also led me to storytelling. As a child and a teenager, I wrote a number of tales and short stories in which he—or some image of him—stood out as a prominent figure. In the 1970s, even though my own alma mater was in a distant city, he found many opportunities to guide my hesitant steps as a medical student with memories and reflections based on his own experience. He kept telling me stories till the end. In the early 1980s, after he had been slowly declining for a couple of years and I suspected he might pass away anytime soon, I asked him to tell me again. This time, I recorded our conversations on tape. I had been well inspired: he died in 1983. Many of his memories were about his training. I later included their transcription in my 2003 book *Plumes d'Ange*, a retelling of his life as a caregiver and a father. Among the many things he taught me, my father always insisted that I should speak English fluently. Since I loved comic books and Westerns, I gladly spent all my teenage summers in England and ended up spending my high school senior year as an exchange student in Bloomington, Minnesota.

When I registered in medical school in Tours, France, in the fall of 1973, I thought I knew pretty well what a doctor was. A doctor looked like a 1930s movie gangster (my dad was a dead ringer for Edward G. Robinson's Little Caesar), *and* he was the kindest person on Earth. A doctor knew an awful lot of complicated things about your body, *and* he could clearly explain to you why you were sick while easing your pain and your fear. A doctor had the biggest and most powerful hands ever, *and* (I witnessed it with my own eyes) he could introduce with the most gentle gestures a terrifyingly long rigid bronchoscope into the mouth of a very sick man lying on his back on an examination table with his head awkwardly tilted backward—and yet cause him no discomfort whatsoever. A doctor could brood over a patient's sufferings, *and* he could still crack the funniest jokes. Whatever happened, a doctor could tell stories that didn't speak ill of people but shared the learning a particular patient had delivered. A doctor learned his life stories from patients. They were his teachers.

I had listened to my father's memories and I had read *Les hommes en blanc* (*The Doctors*), the best-selling medical saga that doctor-writer André Soubiran had published in the late 1940s. I was very much aware that medical training was no piece of cake. But I sincerely thought it would be easy for me to become a doctor: I needed only to remember what kind of man my father was and just follow in his footsteps.

I was such a fool.

In France, between 1973 and 1980, medical education was ghastly, much more so than in Shem's *The House of God*—and not half as funny. French medical schools were then organized pretty much in the likeness of medieval feudal France. My own alma mater, though a public school (there are no private medical schools in this country), was a thoroughly nepotistic institution headed by an unreachable monarch (the dean) ruling over a multitude of small baronies (the specialty wards) in which a self-appointed Elite of Medical Aristocracy (the professors) fiercely fought for their own privileges on a battlefield where nurses, students, and patients alike were as expendable as World War I infantry.

Not unlike India's castes, health care professions were so strictly separated from one another that if you were a midwife, you weren't allowed to train as a medical student, nor the opposite. While I was still a teenager, a brilliant thirty-year-old physicist, who had developed a groundbreaking ultrasound device to measure blood flow, was forced by cardiology professors to take the whole course of medical training before they found him worthy to contribute to patient care with a discovery that is now a standard vascular exploration procedure.

Before 1970, there had been three kinds of medical students in France. The *crème de la crème* were the *internes* (resident doctors), recruited through a grossly unethical century-old process. The students had to memorize strict stereotyped descriptions of diseases and procedures that indulged the current whims and obsessions of the local professors. Each written essay was then read out loud by another student to a triumvirate of potentates who graded it "by ear." Those Chosen Ones, who were eventually dubbed Knights of the Cross, could boast to be the next generation of medical aristocrats. Each professor—who, mind you, had been appointed for life by a small assembly of peers—would someday pick his chief of staff from among the most obedient members of the *crème*. Few of the few might ultimately be entitled to become a professor. Someday. If the current professor ever considered taking time off before his long-awaited demise. And only if his protégé hadn't made any powerful mortal enemies or found out that a younger candidate who happened to be the son of a distinguished colleague had stepped forward in the meantime, in which case the now forty-five-year-old would have no other choice than to leave and set up his own private practice.

Before the 1970s, the *internes* were the only medical students allowed to perform actual clinical procedures on the inpatients—that is, they were the only ones who were *trained* as doctors. And only 10 percent of all medical students became *internes*. The remaining crowd was divided in two other castes: the *externes*, who had also been chosen by an inept selection process and who could fight to do whatever the *internes* were too exhausted or didn't care to do. And the "no-goods," who had failed to pass the *internat* and *externat* exams, were merely allowed . . . to watch. If they could get close enough. In France, up until the late 1960s, one could well become a licensed doctor without having ever cared for—or even made a physical examination of—a single patient.

The May 1968 student protests and workers' strikes brought some change: the *internat* remained untouched, but the "no-good" status disappeared, and all the students attending medical school became *externes* (i.e., second-line trainees) without having to ask for it—provided, of course, that they had survived the painful year (and more often two years) during which you had to sit in overcrowded lecture halls to pass the admission exam. Most of the courses during this time (including math and physics) had nothing to do with medical knowledge and were totally useless for future training. They were only designed as a blade-running tool to get rid of those who didn't bend down far enough on their writing tables. In 1974, the year I passed, 135 students were admitted out of almost 1,000 who had registered. I was number 132. Lucky me: the blade runners hadn't figured out I had actually been sleeping on my math and physics books. But all this had made me really angry—but not gentle.

In my fourth year of medical school, when I finally stepped into a medical ward, I thought I could, at long last, make use of the wisdom and experience my father the doctor had lovingly shared with me. I thought I could shed the anger and learn to be gentle.

Once again, I was such a fool.

Values I thought universal among caregivers had no currency in Tours' university hospital—or in any other French university hospital, as many MDs who were trained in the late 1970s could attest. Doctors discussed patients as if they were cattle, talking down to them. They gave out cruel and crude details to grief-stricken families while keeping crucial information from patients. They made therapeutic decisions without consulting those whose bodies they had decided to cut open or irradiate to a crisp or poison with chemotherapy.

In the 1970s, medical teaching in French university hospitals carried on with the rituals that Charcot and his peers had initiated in the 1890s and that had been institutionalized by one of de Gaulle's secretaries in 1958. In most medical and surgical departments, one professor, appointed for life, ruled—or should I say *reigned*—over care, research, and teaching. Each morning, Monday through Friday, he would enter the ward with the whole staff in his wake. Doctors, residents, interns, nurses, and trainees—a court averaging eight to fifteen people—had to follow *le patron* (the boss) into each room and listen to the comments he uttered without any consideration of privacy in the face of, or his back to, a helpless patient who had no idea he or she was a "medical case." The poor man or woman still had no idea what the situation was when the crowd rushed out of there without showing any intention of listening to the patient's questions, now or ever.

Often, during what was supposed to be the highlight of medical teaching, the professor would run a terrorized *externe* through an ordeal that had less to do with the Socratic method than with Gestapo questioning. To make it short, the professor would harass and humiliate any student who couldn't describe the patient's disease, treatment, and prognosis *before* the externe had had the slightest chance to learn about it. When the student was a woman, *le patron* would eventually make her cry and then unabashedly holler, "What's wrong with you? Do you really expect to ever be a competent doctor if you can't control your own emotions?"

Doctors—mostly males at the time—despised and derided the mostly female nursing staff. Female medical students were openly called *salopes* (whores) by their male counterparts, who complained that these "bitches" were inexcusably robbing some good man of a fine education, since they wouldn't ever practice—nor even graduate—before they got pregnant and married. Wasn't finding a soon-to-be wealthy husband the main reason for any girl to get into medical school, anyway?

Even though family practice was officially praised as the most essential craft in the field of health care, specialized hospital physicians always spoke of family physicians with contempt. They barely answered GPs' mail, and they took every opportunity to let inpatients know that they would be much better off if they stuck with them instead of going back to their country doctor.

Back in the 1970s, lying was the main skill French medical students learned from their elders. Doctors did not only lie to patients; they lied to everyone. They lied to nurses, of course, mostly to terrorize them and get in their pants. They lied to their peers, especially if they didn't agree on a procedure or a diagnosis. They didn't sign their orders or they lied about giving them, so no one could ever put the blame on them if a mistake were made—nurses got nailed for that, too. They lied during their lectures and failed to mention that some distinguished colleague had recently published in a distinguished journal a review that dismissed their own research fancy as totally irrelevant. They lied by making up their own and publishing clinical case stories they had heard from someone else.

They didn't only lie, they drafted inane theories and turned them into truth. France was, and still is, the land of opportunity for hack medical syndromes made up by university professors. Check these few enlightening examples: until the mid-1990s, patients who suffered from typical unilateral pulsatile headaches with nausea weren't diagnosed with migraine, but with so-called liver outbursts (*crises de foie*) and "treated" with gallbladder depurgatory drugs. Women who suffered from panic attacks were stamped as "spasmophiliacs" (whatever that meant) and given magnesium salts. One very imaginative gynecology professor suggested that contraceptive copper IUDs acted by producing a "microscopic inflammatory reaction" in the endometrium and thereby destroyed sperm. Thus, he ruled, no woman with an IUD should ever receive aspirin, steroids, or NSAIDS, lest these drugs' properties compromise the IUD's contraceptive effect and result in unwanted pregnancies. Though the professor's hypothesis was never confirmed, it became a dogma inside the borders of France but of course—and unlike the proverbial Chernobyl radioactive cloud—it didn't catch on abroad. The Belgians, France's immediate neighbors, opened their eyes wide when they heard the story. But to this day, French pharmacists and doctors still pester and scare IUD users with that piece of medical academic fallacy.

Why, you may ask, were so many French professors so incompetent? I could think of at least two explanations: first, their lifelong appointment and total control of the department's activities made them feel all-powerful. And immensely vain. Second, their vanity made them easy prey for the pharmaceutical industry. All the French medical journals at the time were heavily funded by the industry. Drug reps had no qualms about paying for Professor "Dupont's" travels or Professor "Durand's" brand-new car since those distinguished professionals were doing such a great job setting up and publishing conclusive trials with their products. There was not any profit whatsoever in teaching objective evidence-based medicine to medical students. Only in the late 1990s did the French national drug agencies ban unethical funding of medical activities by drug companies.

All this only made me angrier every day.

Fortunately for some of us kids, there were in the Tours medical school very competent teachers and doctors who could teach care and gentleness to those who didn't want to die in anger. They weren't professors, but hard-working physicians and surgeons who much preferred to share with patients and nurses and students rather than dogfight for the top seats. You had to look for them, but they were easy to find, always in the same place—at the patient's side. My mentors Yves Lanson, a urology surgeon; Philippe Bagros, a nephrologist; and Guy Giniès, an ICU specialist, were and still are great teachers and respectful physicians, and I remember very well what I learned from them. Like my father, they were gentle caregivers. But very few of their fellow senior staffers taught the way they did.

Back when I was a twelfth grader at Bloomington's Lincoln High, I had learned to go and get the information where it was: in the library. As a medical student, I had good reasons not to trust what the professors said during their lectures. I went to the library for accurate data. I found out that only a small fraction of my fellow students went to the library and borrowed books or journals. Why would they borrow books, indeed? Nobody suggested they should. Everything they had to learn they could get straight from the horse's—sorry, the professor's—mouth. And one could only borrow *two* books for a period of two weeks, anyway. Besides, most of the French-language medical books were two decades old. The recent ones as well as the only independent (from any funding from the pharmaceutical industry) and reliable journals were in English. Very few of us could read them.

I didn't just read medical books. Ever since spending a year as an exchange student, I had devoured dozens of American short stories and comic books and essays and novels, including any piece that I could lay a hand on written by Isaac Asimov or by William Carlos Williams. Sometime in 1978 or 1979, a lovely Chicago-born Tours bookseller named Nancy urged me to read an American novel she had only one copy of. Said novel had not yet been translated, and I was obviously the only medical student in town she thought could read it and tell her how he felt about it. "You can't go on studying medicine and not read this!" she insisted. I had a crush on Nancy, so I read *The House of God,* and right away I was Roy, and the Fat Man looked like my father, and Berry had Nancy's lovely face. After I finished my reading, I would have kissed Nancy if she hadn't been married. Maybe I should have. She might not have rejected me. After all, this was the 1970s. I had loved the novel and definitely resented the author. Who was *he* to write the kind of book *I* had wanted to pen ever since I had stepped foot in med school, anyway? "Curse you, Red Baron! Damn you, Samuel Shem!" I yelled. But *The House of God* definitely helped me ease my ever-growing anger with insane laughter. And it suggested there were means for me to strike right back at what I endured.

In 1983, one year after I graduated from medical school, I joined the writing staff of *La revue Prescrire,* the first independent drug bulletin in France. A monthly magazine, it had been created only three years before. During the next six years, I discovered that most of what I had been told in med school about drugs and therapeutics dated back to the prewar era. Everything I needed to know about evidence-based medicine, clinical trials, and scientific thinking I learned while I worked at *Prescrire.* Its staff was a motley crew of merry men who had one thing in common: they didn't want to keep eating the crap they'd been fed in medical school. They wanted to be and to train competent caregivers.

While at *Prescrire,* I read and reviewed English-written medical journals and wrote many articles based on those readings. One of my most important papers, around 1985, was a review of guidelines on morphine prescription for cancer pain. Cancer pain was not treated in France at the time. French patients had to wait until 1996, when a secretary of health decided it was time for all French medical students to learn how to prescribe painkillers.

At the time I joined the staff of *Prescrire,* I became a country doctor, and for the next decade, I held a practice in a very small village in Sarthe—deep, deep rural France. A few years later, I was one of the cofounders of the local Balint group. Pierre Bernachon, our supervisor, had learned his craft with Michael and Enid Balint in the early 1960s. Although he had been trained as a pediatrician, he had always practiced as a GP and had become one of the most respected physician-writers of his time and one of the rare Balint supervisors who had not undergone psychoanalysis. He was a fine teacher and a good man.

My experiences, blunders, and colorful encounters as a Balintian physician gave birth to a personal project: in the last pages of each issue of *Prescrire,* I published reflections on my everyday practice along with similar contributions sent by other writing doctors. Many readers thanked us because each month, when the new issue showed up in their mailbox, they read those pages first: there, fellow physicians shared their feelings about common mishaps and hardships. The last pages of *Prescrire* were a place where being a doctor was much more than just scribbling down prescriptions. Contributions came from all over France; they dealt with the doctor-patient relationship and professional solidarity, issued calls for the profession to resist the industry's siren songs, and shared clinical insights and readings.

I left *Prescrire* in 1989 just after I published my first novel, *La vacation,* based on my experience in an abortion clinic. For several years after that, I was a medical consultant for health magazines. The guys I worked with were amazed that this MD was willing to explain illnesses and medical procedures in simple, intelligible terms to their readership. They just weren't used to that. I didn't know how else to do it: my father and mentors had trained me that way.

Since I could not only read English but also—thanks to my *Prescrire* years— write decent medical papers, I started to translate American medical literature. Soon, medical publishers trusted me to edit translations of huge treaties— *Harrison's Principles of Internal Medicine* and such. I found out with horror that many self-proclaimed "translators" didn't know what they were doing. Most of them were specialized attending physicians who had little or no knowledge of the English language and even less knowledge of evidence-based medicine and scientific writing. Many translations of medical treatises were thus badly flawed—to say the least. And since few people in the publishing companies could edit them, they often went into print uncorrected. How could medical students who did not read English get accurate information from these?

In 1993, I left my private practice and started earning a living as a translator for several years and worked part time in the hospital's family planning clinic. I did brood over the loss of my work as a country doctor. So I started to write about it and seized the opportunity to poke fun at the medical education I had received. I sat down and wrote a case study—in reverse. These were sufferings of a country doctor, Dr. Bruno Sachs, observed by his patients.

My father had taught me to be a listener. In the clinic, I still listened to women's narratives. Thanks to our Balint group, I had learned not to confuse my own fears with those of my patients. I had learned to appreciate their stories as *stories.* And when I started telling stories of my own, I didn't need to make much effort to remember tears and fears, grief and denial, and I used them to dress up my characters.

In 1998, a few months after it was published, *La maladie de Sachs* (*The Case of Dr. Sachs*) had sold over 250,000 copies in France alone. The general public loved it. Many readers came to me or wrote saying they now understood what being a doctor was and how tricky it sounded to make sense of patients' complaints. Many added that they felt relieved: if, as the book suggested, Bruno Sachs understood his patients, their own doctor could understand them too. In fact, dozens of doctors—especially GPs—were given the book as presents by grateful patients. And I can't tell you how many fellow physicians came to me, saying, "This book describes my practice, my patients! How did you do that?" Others came laughing because on several instances, a patient was reading the book in the waiting room, and they, too, had a copy on their desk, and they ended up discussing the patient-doctor relationship described in one of Dr. Bruno Sachs's encounters.

One line in the novel became especially popular among the general public: "Know the difference between God and a doctor? God doesn't pretend he's a doctor." I had heard the line in an early *Law & Order* episode. But it sounded so much like something Roy Basch or the Fat Man might have said that I had to put it in my novel.

I wish my father had been alive. I would have loved to share those stories with him.

And I wish he had been alive in 2004, when I published *Les trois médecins* (*The Three Doctors*), a novel based on my medical school years. At the time I read *The House of God,* in the late 1970s, I was sadly convinced I wasn't good enough to be a doctor *and* a writer.

For the next thirty years I dreamed of writing an adventure novel that would also be the story of a friendship, the account of students' political struggles in the 1970s, a dramatic love story, and a sizzling description of medical training in late twentieth-century France. The project was so ambitious I decided I couldn't achieve it. Nobody could. Well, Samuel Shem had, but he was just another damn American writer! He was born in the midst of John Dos Passos, Isaac Asimov, William Carlos Williams, Stan Lee, and Jack Kirby. These guys had it made.

Then the success of *Sachs* helped me overcome that feeling, and I thought I should go back to read *The House of God* again. Maybe it would help. It didn't. How could I ever hope to even remotely emulate that! I could see the Fat Man grin at me. *Curse you, Red Baron! Damn you, Samuel Shem!*

Then, one miraculous day, I suddenly realized that, in fact, one classic French adventure novel successfully mixed politics, love, friendship, and professional training: Alexandre Dumas's *The Three Musketeers.*

You know writers. As far as delusions of grandeur go, they're even worse than doctors. If Leonard Bernstein and Jerome Robbins could remake *Romeo and Juliet* into *West Side Story,* couldn't I remake Dumas's novel into a medical epic set in the fictitious city of Tourmens during the 1970s?

Nobody said I couldn't. And, frankly, I didn't ask.

I turned meek King Louis XIII into Fisinger, the dean of medicine married to Sonia, a strong feminist hematologist who performed illegal abortions with the help of her British lover, George Buckley. Cardinal Richelieu became Deputy Dean Leriche, an ob-gyn who viewed women as underlings; he had two sidekicks—Rochefort and Milady—who fought to become his chief of staff; their *internes* were modern-day cardinal's guards. André, Basile, and Christophe, three idealistic med students sworn to become family physicians, were my own heroic Musketeers. Young Bruno Sachs, a newcomer in Tourmens medical school, took over d'Artagnan's part.

I grinned back at the Fat Man. Finally, I had found a way to channel the anger against French medical institutions that had been brewing inside me for thirty years into the fun ride of a handful of gentle coed souls—There are sex-craving free-riding female *Med*sketeers in my novel!—who wanted to become caregivers.

Les trois médecins did pretty well. Then came the biggest surprise. For the last few years, many teenagers had started med school after reading *The Case of Dr. Sachs*, and some teachers in med school all over France had made the book required reading for their courses on medical ethics. In 2005, I started to receive letters from students who had gone on to read *Les trois médecins* as well. Many of those—the most striking pieces have been posted on my Website—boiled with frustration. "Thirty years have gone by," they wrote, "and yet the horrible things you have witnessed as a student and eventually turned into an epic narrative are still going on. French medical schools are still a place where patients are not cared for, where students are despised, and where nepotism reigns." I had a hard time believing it. I thought things had changed. I thought French medical education, although it was a late bloomer, had finally gotten on the right track. I couldn't believe that the worst things I remembered from thirty years ago were still happening today.

Again, I was a fool. I found that out a few months ago.

In 2006, I had been working for the Department of Family Practice in one of Paris's medical schools and was assigned to teach such classes as How to Give a Bad Piece of News to a Patient and How to Deal with a Difficult Patient to young *externes*. That year, a television producer who had read *Les trois médecins* approached me to work on a documentary. She wanted to show how young people become doctors in France nowadays. I outlined the project with her, and we brought our proposal to my colleagues at the Department of Family Practice and to the dean. They all thought it was a bright idea. Filming took place for several months in the 2006–7 academic year. Thanks to the dean's support and with his blessing, talented film director Marie Agostini followed a handful of students and attending physicians along the corridors of several Parisian university medical wards.

A few weeks before its May 2007 airing on Arte, I screened all ten thirty-minute episodes of *L'école de médecine* over a weekend. I thought I was being pulled back thirty-five years in the past. I found out that today in Paris, professors still enter tiny rooms with a dozen people in their wake, stand at the bedside of muted patients, and, in full-frontal vanity, humiliate despairing students who can't describe in full detail surgical procedures nobody knows about. Scared-to-shit *externes* are still left alone when they draw femoral blood for the first time from hemiplegic patients. Patients' diagnoses and imminent lethal prognoses are still unabashedly discussed in corridors while the patients themselves have not yet been given the information. *"By the way, should we tell her? She might want to go and spend her last days with her kids. . . . Naaa . . . Why bother?"* And professors still make female students cry and still shout, "What's wrong with you?"

I can see the Fat Man grin again.

I guess my anger isn't going to wane anytime soon.

Justice, Virtue, and
the Laws of The House of God

Justice and Humor in The House of God

MARTHA ELKS AND ISAAC M. T. MWASE

The House of God by Samuel Shem documents well, in its own twisted way, the challenges and conflicts of internal medicine residency in the United States in the 1970s. Twisted in its preoccupation with sex, the story is irreverently funny, treating every character simultaneously with compassion and with contempt. Cynical humor and exaggeration certainly dominate the story, but justice is a strong undercurrent. It is the conjunction of a variety of injustices that form the impetus and the underlying motivation for the ongoing expression of aggression as humor. These injustices include the exploitation of the interns in overwork, the role of hierarchies over competence in the power structure of the hospital, inequities in roles and power in the health care team, and the glaring inequities in treatment and economic status. There are also injustices in the hidden barriers of access that lurk just beneath the surface of the story—discrimination against Jewish physicians that was the basis for the foundation of the House of God and the discrimination that African American physicians face. By the end of the story, the protagonist finds that while humor and his friends have helped him survive, he must escape the absurdities of internal medicine to recover himself.

The House of God tells of a time before AIDS, before DRGs, before managed care and controlled lengths of stay, before hour limits for residents. It was at the start of women's entry into medicine in large numbers as integration of the professions and other workplaces gathered momentum. In humorous and surrealistic episodes, it pulls back the hospital gown to reveal an interesting truth: since physicians and other health care delivery professionals really cannot conquer death (or even disease), their enemies are the patients and the system. The best treatment for sick patients is doing as little as possible when doing more leads to serious medical complications.

As a documentary, the book accurately depicts the suffering intrinsic to becoming a doctor. It alludes to the first two phases of suffering—the force-feeding of information in the preclinical courses and the hierarchical hazing of students on the wards and clinics. It depicts well the many conflicts that the interns face—that the science they are taught and the agendas of their supervisors have little relationship to the wants and needs of their patients. If anything, the book underplays the very real overwork, sleep deprivation, and myriad conflicts of interest that characterize hospital-based residency training. It would be wonderful to report that it is inaccurate in its presentation of self-centered supervisory physicians, punitive hierarchies, differences in the treatment of rich and poor, physicians' failure to perceive the patients' needs, and denial of the human frailties of the faculty and house staff—but those are the portions of the book that show more truth than falsehood. The cynical humor of the physicians is too close to the truth of the experience of house staff then and now. It is one of the few tools that the physicians have to deal with the absurdity of overwork and competing demands.

In order to understand this story of interns in internal medicine training, it is useful to understand a derogatory term that does not appear in the book. Physicians trained as internists are known as "fleas," as in "All over their patients like fleas." Surgeons use this term to show disdain for the internists, who are too thorough, too detailed, who know too much. It is a mark of the psychology of the internist that many embrace this term with pride, deeply convinced that completeness, comprehensiveness, and attention to detail are necessary for optimal decision making and management in the care of hospitalized patients.

As an exposé of life in a teaching hospital, *The House of God* to nonmedical eyes is a terrifying tale about the crass treatment of patients. To an intern, a patient is a gomer or a candidate to be turfed to another department in the hospital specialty system. It is understandably horrifying to see the chaos, complexity, and incoherence that are intrinsic to hospital care, especially in a training setting. In general, American medicine has done a good job of hiding (or failing to communicate clearly about) the risks and limitations of hospital-based care. Amid this chaos, good outcomes randomly come to the rich or the poor, with a major role played by chance and happenstance, and little or no role played by physician competence—a justice of chance, not of intent. Through a variety of characters in *The House of God*—Berry, Roy, the Fat Man, Chuck, the Leggo, the Fish, Molly, Eat My Dust Eddie, Wayne Potts, Harold "the Runt" Runtsky, Dr. Davis, Nate Zock, Sergeant Gilheeny, Officer Quick, and the many other fascinating characters—one comes to appreciate the absurdities of hospital-based health care.

Some elements of the book that are thought of as original to the author are instead artful presentation of house staff culture of the time. The terminology, the black humor, the underlying sense that (some) patients and the hospital leadership are the enemy—these were a widespread part of American medical house staff culture in the 1970s. "Turfed" and "buffed" were in wide use before the book was published. Sexual medical banter was an integral part of (male) communication that has since significantly withered with the influx of women in medicine (rising from about 5–10 percent to about 50 percent). The work dances around some truths we are reluctant to acknowledge in Western culture and Western medicine—our learning and science cannot conquer death. While one may be seduced into a medical career with the vision of being a crusader fighting death and disease, what one finds when one peels back the covers is that both of these have us beat, regardless of the weapons that one brings to bear. In denial about this defeat, we turn our aggression to each other, the patient, the system, and so forth. There is humor in these turns. Directly in punitive but pragmatic hierarchies, indirectly in passive aggression, sideways in humor, indirectly in sexual aggression and fantasy, overtly in affirmative action practices, covertly in lingering prejudices and social stratification, we play out our fighting energies in denial of death. In these fights we find our humanity and discover meaning in life. Each character in the book is a case study in how to grapple with the challenges posed by pain and suffering. The interns use humorous distancing from their patients to keep themselves from the kind of severe emotional drainage that might lead to suicide. The hospital training hierarchy and the house staff are a portrait of a physician training system that the interns see as in dire need of an overhaul if the demands of justice as fairness are to be satisfied. Each character finds ways to cope with a badly broken and intern-breaking system.

CHARACTER STUDIES

Roy Basch: The King of Interns

The narrator of the book, Roy Basch, experiences a transformation during the year of internship. We see through his eyes the glorious yet terrifying honor of being an intern at the House of God—a Jewish hospital built in part to address the discrimination against Jewish medical students and interns. "The House of God had been founded in 1913 by the American people of Israel when their medically qualified sons and daughters could not get good internships at good hospitals because of discrimination" (Shem, *House*, 1978 21). This background of discrimination is an undercurrent that underlies the rest of the book—as several key characters have been affected by discrimination such as that which stimulated the building of the House of God.

Starting with the expected anxieties of the new intern, Roy worries that he will not be good enough, as in a discussion with Berry:

"Help, hellllp," I said.
"Roy, you really are in bad shape."

"How bad is it?"

"Bad. Last week I hospitalized a patient who was found curled up under the covers just like that, and he was less anxious than you."

"Can you hospitalize me?"

"Do you have insurance?"

"Not till I start the internship."

"Then you'd have to go to the State Facility."

"What should I do? I've tried everything, and I'm still scared to death." (23)

Thus, in the first few pages of the book we are already confronting the injustices of discrimination and the injustice of the role of insurance in America for access to needed health care services (and the injustice of linking insurance to employment as we do in America). The protagonist deals with the absurdities he encounters through passive aggression ("faking" the testing and evaluation of the patients), humor, and fantasy of sexual conquest. He has several helpful guides along the way—especially the Fat Man in the hospital and Berry outside the hospital. The Fat Man gives him the lessons straightup.

> Again, like the day before, most of what I'd learned at the BMS about medicine either was irrelevant or wrong. Thus, for a dehydrated Ina, hydration made her worse. The treatment for depression was to order a barium enema, and the treatment for Potts's third admission, a man with pain in his abdomen but who "knew all of you doctors are Nazis but I'm not quite sure just yet which one of you is Himmler," was not a barium enema and bowel run, but what the Fat Man called a "TURF TO PSYCHIATRY."
>
> "What's a TURF?"
>
> "To TURF is to get rid of, to get off your service and onto another, or out of the House altogether. Key concept. It's the main form of treatment in medicine." (58–59)

Confronted with an impossible level of work and having to cure incurables, the only way to save oneself is to identify a reason to send incurable patients to someone else, to make them someone else's problem. To "turf" them.

In another instance, Fats advises lying in the chart. Also, the priorities of the internist-diagnostician—to be systematic and accurate in diagnosis through the use of extensive and invasive testing, as needed—prove to be causes of problems in and of themselves. "First, do no harm" is not a strong value in the context of the need to be comprehensive and accurate and rule out unlikely possibilities, as Roy's supervising resident, Jo, tries to get him to do in accordance with standard medical practice. Avoiding doing the medical testing he learned in medical school, Roy finds that avoiding the tests but making the chart look good is the key to good care. "Sure, continue the work-up in purely imaginary terms. BUFF the chart with the imaginary results of the imaginary test, Anna will recover to her demented state, the work-up will show no treatable cause for it, and everybody's happy. Nothing to it" (105).

The distasteful recognition of the patient as enemy is a secret trauma for most physicians. Physicians do not wish to acknowledge this, but at some point in training the patient becomes dehumanized as a fascinating case, or as the cause of their own sense of impotence. Physicians deal with these traumas through the very key observation of the book—THE PATIENT IS THE ONE WITH THE DISEASE. The messianic complex of the physician that encourages him or her to take responsibility for the patient's disease is a true recipe for failure and suicide. Fats, depicted as a cynical resident at the start of the book, provides the insight and truth that help Roy come to this realization. This recognition allows him, by the end of the book, to detach himself from the battle and to have sympathy for the others still caught up in the struggle.

Roy confronts his own feelings of inadequacy in confronting the injustice faced by his patients and their family members and the impotence of modern medicine in providing help and answers. In working with a patient in the emergency ward, he struggles with a patient in pain.

> "Damn you, look at her, she's suffering, Now you gotta give her something for her pain." I said I would not. I went back to the nursing station to write up my findings. The boyfriend pursued me, and although the woman was embarrassed and stood near the door wanting to leave, he would not, and began to see the crowded E.R. as a forum: "Goddamn you. I knew we wouldn't get any help here. You just want her to suffer, 'cause you enjoy it. You honkies don't give a shit, as long as we get the hell out." My temper rose, and I felt that warm limbic flush creeping about my ears, my neck. I wanted to jump the counter and beat the shit out of him, or have him beat the shit out of me. He couldn't have known that I shared his sense of being a victim, his sense of despair about the wrecking of black women by forces out of control, his frustration with disease, with life. I even had grown to share his paranoia. I couldn't tell him, and he couldn't hear. (242)

Roy can recognize the injustices around him and for him and is furious. Unable to resolve them with work or learning, he continues to defuse them with humor, numbing himself to the pain and losing himself.

Humor is part of the aikido technique that helps him to slip out of the fight to cure, to the true needs underlying the struggle. He does grow to be a better doctor than his teacher. Fats remains a cynical practitioner using technique but without apparent true heart. Roy, on the other hand, comes to realize the necessity of reconnecting with his humanity to be a good physician.

> I finally realized what all these conjunctions meant: hope. What was my hope now? To take a year off, to risk, grow, be with others, even to be with parents who'd loved me despite my shabby treatment of them, through so many arrogant years. Was the Fat Man my hope any longer? In what he'd taught me, yes, in showing me to one truly great American Medical Invention: the creation of a foolproof system that took sincere energetic guys and, with little effort, turned them into dull, grandiose docs who could live with the horror of disease and the deceit of "cure," who could "go with" the public's fantasy of the right to perfect health devoid of even the deterioration of age, a whole nation of Hyper Hoopers and other Californians who expected the day to be sunny, the body young, to be surfing along always on the waves of vitality, and who, when the clouds come, the marriage fails, the erection wilts, the brown blotches of age break out like geriatric acne on the backs of the hands, in terror, wipe out. (406–7)

In the end, however, he chooses to escape to a year off and psychiatry. Helped by Berry to realize his pain, he knows he has to reclaim himself.

> Later, Berry welcomed me back to her, and I felt her caring arms around me as if for the first time. Awakening, I began to thaw. I began to feel a little, then a rush of feeling that was scary and overwhelming. Choked up, I began to talk. On and into the night. I talked about the things I'd blotted out. The theme, over and over, coating my bedroom with a grayish-white mottled skin, was death. I talked about the horror of the dying, and the horror of the dead. (360)

There is a lack of narrative coherence in the work in the award to Roy at the end. In spite of the truth of his insights, his recognition as the "Most Valuable Intern"—even that Roy would care about such an award from such a morally contorted system—is not plausible. Roy clearly confronted the system's deficits and refused to play the academic game of research-based one-upmanship. These are the traits that would have been rewarded in this system, and these are the skills and traits that Roy learns are hollow and meaningless. The recognition by Zock also hits a false note. While Zock would have liked the courage shown by Roy toward the Zock family and in his speaking the truth, he would well have understood the inexperience and naïveté intrinsic in this intern and would not have thumbed his nose at the system in this way. These rewards do add to the recognition of the courage needed to walk away from all this as he did at the end. Truly, recognizing the need to leave and making the change underscore the major transformation Roy has made.

Roy, helped by others, finds that there is no equilibrium for him in internal medicine, takes time off, and plans to continue training later in psychiatry, an area in which he sees himself being able to practice as a whole person, not walled off against injustice, against his own impotence to really help his patients.

Chuck's Justice

A backdrop of *The House of God* was the changing racial composition of all professions. Chuck is the character in the book who refracts some of the issues of integration in the late 1970s. He is Roy's best friend, if one can ever have such a friend during the dehumanizing year of an internship. Chuck is black. He is from Memphis. Throughout his internship, a shot of some Jack Daniels seems always within reach from the black bag he is always carrying. He is the quintessential black professional, made to feel an additional sense of inadequacy simply because he is black. Roy realizes that those who regard Chuck as a charity case are wrong. Chuck has a sensitivity and intelligence that are severely tested and nearly crushed, but his sophisticated self-determination suggests that a resurrection will occur from the death induced by the horrors of his House of God internship.

The road from Memphis to the House of God was not easy. This may sound preposterous to say about someone who gets the internship in part because he is black. But the character we encounter in *The House of God* is not merely an affirmative action physician. He has every right to the internship. Though unorthodox in his appearance, his demeanor, and his lifestyle, he exemplifies a coping mechanism that leaves him at the end of the internship with that spark ignitable by a vision of a reformed and reforming medical practice. Up until the end of the House of God internship, Chuck has lived in response to other people's initiative. In fact that pattern might continue if at the end of his internship year he accepts the invitation to become an officer at the National Institutes of Health. For the first time, in response to such invitation, he declines. Chuck is poised to head south: "I figure I gone about as white as I can go. . . . Tomorrow mornin'. Back to Memphis. Back home. . . . But I'm gonna try. I'm gonna get back in shape, find a black woman, be a regular old black doc with a lotta money and a big bad lim-O-zeene. And that'll jes' about do it for old me" (Shem, *House,* 2003 373).

"Fill out and return this card." By acting according to this instruction in materials from Oberlin College, the University of Chicago Medical School, and the internship at the House of God, Chuck set his life itinerary accordingly. Though he confesses to a youngster's desire to join the army, there is some ambivalence at the beginning of Chuck's medical internship because he really wanted to be a singer. And Chuck can sing.

Chuck is a symbol of endurance in the book. Roy likes him for the very reason that Chuck is a survivor. Chuck becomes for Roy and for the book a signature human statement that one can have humble beginnings, have life throw the worst one can expect from it, and still emerge with a humorous humanity and a profound hope for the future. The first day of the internship depicts much that is humorous about Chuck and his sense of identity. He arrives dressed like a mugger. Why? "'Cause, you see, in Chicago where I come from, there are only two kinds of dudes—the muggers and the mugged. Now, if you don't dress like a mugger, man, you automatically gets yourself mugged. You dig?" (28). Chuck's self-representation is deliberate. Therein is his genius. He knows how to be a shrewd chameleon, able to blend into its surroundings so that it can find prey, while avoiding being prey to other predators. When it suits him, he comes across as untutored, ignorant, and an abuser of the English language. When push comes to shove, he has reservoirs of resources to dismantle racist assessments of his character and competency as a physician or even on the basketball court. A rebel among rebels, Chuck hears but refuses to listen to the Fish when the chief resident decries the Memphis intern's dirty whites and unbuttoned shirt without a tie. The same episode occurs with the female resident Jo. His "Fine, fine" is an acknowledgement of the power dynamics of the House of God but is also dismissive of authority. Chuck's dress code never improves. Add the Jack Daniels, and it actually gets worse and worse.

While Roy manages to survive the internship because of people who care for him, including Chuck, his friend draws from deep internal resources in addition to their budding friendship. "While I had Fats . . . Chuck had himself" (95). Chuck, however, nurtured an off-duty camaraderie with Roy that certainly contributed to the resilience that helped him stumble to the finishing line of his internship year at the House of God. Roy is the yin, and Chuck the yang: "But we used each other—him using me for the facts and the numbers and me using him for the nuts and bolts—and we risked, and we learned" (99). The team they forge for their medical internship is also apparent on the basketball court. Both love the game. They go at each other and jointly at others two out of every three nights. As they get to know each other playing basketball, watching the game on TV while drinking some bourbon, and generally hanging out together, Roy comes to discover a truth about Chuck that is often true of victims of racism: "My new friend's studied indifference was only and all an act" (100). Such is the camaraderie between Roy and Chuck; they cover for each other in taking care of difficult patients, care that often takes the form of turfing and buffing their gomers. It is a hilarious scene that sets up such mutuality: "I turned and saw Chuck and the Runt, kneeling on the tile floor, looking up at me like cocker spaniel pups in the window of a pet shop" (176).

When Chuck's true colors as an excellent player emerge during a basketball game against one particularly nasty and arrogant medical student, Roy asks him to explain his pretensions. Chuck's response could be given by highly successful blacks in the professions and in academia: "If'n you let on what you are and who you are and what you got and how someone can use you, you get yourself used worse. . . . I may be painin', man, but nobody's gonna know it. Being cool is the only way of stayin' alive" (101–2).

The reader is never completely sure whether Chuck is a shrewd intern who plays dumb, or whether he is a consummate con artist. He cannot be anything but shrewd. His smarts are not derived from books. Chuck's knowledge is from doing. He is the quintessence of experimental medicine. It does not seem that we are expected to believe him when Chuck credits his knowledge to anything other than reading: "See, I never read nuthin'. I just did it all" (41). However he gains insight into medical problems, he demonstrates his genius by being more often than not right in diagnoses of disease and the appropriate therapies for such diseases. His counsel to Wayne Potts is that a particular patient be given steroids. This patient becomes the Yellow Man and a factor in the unraveling of Potts, who did not pay any attention to Chuck's diagnosis and treatment recommendation.

The incident with the Broccoli Lady is what transforms Chuck in the eyes of all of the House of God from "a dumb black admitted on quota" to "a smart tern" (129). A patient who would become the Broccoli Lady comes into Chuck's care, unable to breathe. She has already been in the care of the interns Howard and Mad Dog and an attending, Putzel. Chuck famously examines "this whale." He decides to look inside her mouth. He spies some broccoli jammed in the throat of this foul-smelling lady who is not breathing. Simply through uncommon common sense, Chuck saves the life of the Broccoli Lady.

There is hardly an intern in the House of God who is not highly sexed. Chuck is no exception. The early suggestion in the book is that he gets his sex from the boss of bed making, a big Cuban woman named Hazel. Getting this sexual satisfaction also ensures Chuck and his fellow interns clean sheets on the beds interns use for what little sleep they can get when they are on call at night. Though they engage in doublespeak, you are left without any doubt later in the book that the relationship between Chuck and Hazel is "real hot and red":

> "You got your hot water and clean sheets, Chuck?"
> "Great, Hazel, just great, gurl. Thanks."
> "And your car? Maybe it needs some fixing?"

"Oh, yeah, Hazel, my car's not runnin' well. Needs a lotta work. Gotta get my car fixed for sure, soon. See, my front end needs some looking at. Yeah, that's it, my front end."

"Front end? Ho! You bad boy! And when do you want to put your car in the garage?"

"Well, let's see—tomorrow, gurl, how about tomorrow?"

"OK," said Hazel, giggling. "Tomorrow. Front end? Ba'boy. *Adios*." (104)

You get a glimpse of Chuck as a mentor and an alpha male in his relationship with Towl—"Towl? Towl, boy, you get in here stat!" yelled Chuck. Towl is a four-foot tall BMS "with thick black glasses and thick black skin, with a voice gruff as a drill sergeant's and a vocabulary that was short and tough like him" (107). Chuck assesses Towl as the "best damn BMS you ever saw." He is certainly at his best humorous self when Chuck asks him to describe patients under his and his superior intern's care: "Rhhmmmmm rhmmmm twenty-two patients: eleven gommers, five sickees, and six turkeys who nevah shoulda been heah in the foist place. All in all, nine of 'em are on da rolla costa" (108).

Chuck is no saint. He contributes equally generously with Roy to the sexual debauchery of the once shy and retiring Runtsky. He and Roy persuade a nurse named Angel to go all out in destroying the Runt's sexual inhibitions. She does break them down all right. "I've been fucking my eyes out," said the Runt (125). The sexual escapades are between consenting adults, and, in a pre-HIV world, relatively harmless, but a slide into alcoholism threatens to destroy Chuck. His alcoholism becomes clearly noticeable to Berry and Roy when the three attend a party hosted by the Leggo. He gets smashed. When he and Roy manage to drive erratically and amazingly safely to the House of God, they get to assess their drinking bout at the Leggo's party:

> "So Berry's a little worried about me, huh?" asked Chuck.
> "Yup. More than a little. Hey, I'm worried about you too."
> "Well, Roy, tell you a little secret: so am I, man, so am I." (Shem, *House*, 1978 236)

Chuck's slide into alcoholism is accompanied by less and less attention to physical health. He becomes fatter and out of shape. His relationship with Roy becomes increasingly bland and even chilly. He retreats into his self-protective shell with the habitual "Fine, fine" (Shem, *House*, 2003 261). Fine he is not. The disintegration comes to a head with the suicide death of Potts. This forces Chuck to try to salvage his supportive friendship with Roy. He is the one who comes to Roy's aid when deep psychosis and paranoia threaten to push the MVI (most valuable intern) over the edge.

Chuck eventually comes to terms with his life's purpose. He comes to the realization that one year of interning at the House of God was enough for him. If he had not clung together in disillusionment with Roy, Hooper, Eddie, and the Runt, he would not have come to the decision to switch to a residency in psychiatry. "No foolin', Chief. What this country needs is a high-class black shrink, right?" (351).

Berry the Savior

But for Berry, it is doubtful that Roy Basch successfully completes the House of God internship in internal medicine. She is a gravitational love force that keeps Roy from unraveling. She opens and closes the book. She is the central character by which all the other women in Roy's life find definition. Roy's resident Jo is clueless about the sexuality of House of God interns, whereas Berry is the quintessence of an understanding love. Her love for Roy comes into sharp focus against the backdrop of bohemian sexualities suggested in various characters, including Molly, Angel, and Hazel.

It is Berry's love for Roy that helps him navigate the treacherous aspects of his internship. Even though their relationship comes close to breaking, Berry valiantly fights to save it. She wins. They end up headed for the altar. Love triumphs over death.

Berry is a clinical psychologist. She reads Freud. Her powers of assessment and her clinical psychological recommendations help Roy deal with the serious challenges that arise at several critical moments of his internship. When Roy is scared to death at the start of his internship, Berry's recommendation is denial. Like a mother and her child on the first day of school, Berry deposits Roy at the House of God, ushers him out of her car, and presses a note into his hand: "Meet you here at five P.M. Good luck. Love, Berry" (16). As Roy grapples with various aspects of his internship, Berry is there genuinely trying to understand the whole experience and its impact on their fragile relationship. Their relationship had survived their years at the BMS.

It is with Berry that Roy seeks to establish a role for humor in his dealings with death at the House of God, as in this interchange in which Berry admonishes Roy:

> "Laughing at this Ina is sick."
> "It does seem sick right now, but it didn't then."
> "Why did you laugh at her?"
> "I don't know. It was hilarious at the time."
> "I'd like to understand. Try again."
> "Nope. I can't." (64)

Berry expresses her displeasure with Roy and the Fat Man for laughing at their patients. Roy confesses to Berry that he actually does not want to laugh at his patients but has to if he is to deal with what he perceives as their intent to hurt him:

> "Yeah. They killed me."
>
> "Who did?"
>
> "The gomers. But the Fat Man just told me that they hurt everybody and that's modern medicine so I don't know what to think anymore. He said to trash my illusions and the world would beat a pathway to my door." (83)

Freud becomes the prism through which Berry seeks to understand Roy's pain and her own. When they experience a relationship on the rocks (ROR), Berry has to find a way of dealing with Roy's infidelity. The ROR is induced by Roy's relationship with Molly. They do it often whenever he is at the House of God. Berry interprets these escapades as the unfolding of Roy's primary processes according to Freud's pleasure principle. When Roy finds out that Berry already knows about his flings with Molly, he has to swallow his jealousy when she assures him that what is good for the gander is good for the goose: "We'll keep this love going, Roy, I'm going to fight for it. Just remember, though—your freedom means my freedom too. OK, Buddy?" (209).

Berry's analysis of Roy yields nuggets of wisdom for coping with the challenges of an internship at the House of God. She urges Roy to "survive to bear witness, to record the ones who didn't survive" (Shem, *House*, 1978 362). Her talk therapy helps Roy realize that it is the relationships that he has with others connected to the House of God—Gilheeny, Quick, Cohen, Chuck, the Runt, and others—that keep him going.

Berry saves the day for Roy through her masterful assessment of his House of God experiences. She helps Roy deal with his cynicism, paranoia, and anger. Her diagnosis of his condition at various points in the internship is on target. When Roy enters a phase where he stews with rage, Berry says: "You've got to be socialized all over again, Roy. No one can be that angry and be in this world with anyone else. Your friends are really worried about you" (Shem, *House*, 2003 224).

The Fat Man's Humor

The Fat Man is the quintessential "slick" in training. "Slick" is a derogatory term that comes from the time of crafty community physicians who abused the house staff by smoothly communicating with the patients to engender a sense of trust and dedication and then relying on the work of the house staff to take care of the patient and do the needed tests and evaluation. The community physician would then reap the appreciation of patients for the hard work of the residents. It was like a slick con game where the house staff did the work and the community physician got the money and the glory for the care given. Putzel is such an individual, described in the book as "the hand-holder from the suburbs" (Shem, *House,* 1978 42). Fats has learned to work this system and shares his insights with Roy. Key skills are hand-holding and the use of testing to have the desired impact on the patient, not for medical reasons. Fats's skills at hand-holding are illustrated in his interaction with Dr. Sanders, a patient with advanced cancer. "The Fat Man, a jolly green blimp in his surgical pajamas, floated in, and with a few words with Dr. Sanders established a marvelous rapport. A warmth filled the room, a trust, a plea to help, a promise to try" (93).

As to the "therapeutic" use of testing, Fat Man tells Roy early on to use unnecessary testing for its psychological impact on the patients.

> "What is it with this GI workup?" I asked. "She says she's depressed and has a headache."
>
> "It's the specialty of the House," said Fats, "the bowel run. TTB—Therapeutic Trial of Barium."
>
> "There's nothing therapeutic about barium. It's inert."
>
> "Of course it is. But the bowel run is the great equalizer."
>
> "She's depressed. There's nothing wrong with her bowels."
>
> "Of course there's not. There's nothing wrong with her, either. It's just that she got tired of going to Putzel's office, and he got tired of calling at her house, so they both pile into his white Continental and come to our House. She's fine, she's LOL in NAD—a Little Old Lady in No Apparent Distress. You don't think Putzel knows that too? And every time he holds Sophie's hand, it's forty of your Blue Cross dollars. Millions." (42)

Part of this outcomes-focused patient management involves the "buffing" of the chart—lying and providing misleading documentation to prevent the ordering and performing of risky and potentially harmful medical tests while the patient recovers from her problem. "Sure, continue the work-up in purely imaginary terms. BUFF the chart with the imaginary results of the imaginary test, Anna will recover to her demented state, the work-up will show no treatable cause for it, and everybody's happy. Nothing to it" (105).

Although the Fat Man is a very important guide for Roy as he learns to "do more by doing less," he is a limited teacher, for his career goal is to be gastroenterologist to the stars, to parlay his confident manner, insight, and interpersonal skills—not into health improved or lives saved but into high income and prestige. He can deliver Roy from being eaten alive by the system like Potts, but he cannot help him to find his own buried resources.

Sergeant Gilheeny and Officer Quick

They appear in *The House of God* always together. They are the emergency room policemen. But they are more than that. They become seers. They see and understand what their more educated intern associates cannot. Their insights are drawn from a continuing education curriculum of their own creation. Whenever they are on shift, they mine the wealth of knowledge embedded in the brilliant minds of each successive wave of new interns. It is almost eerie the way they are able to anticipate events. They become a source of stability and a navigational reference point for MVI Roy and his cohort.

Gilheeny and Quick join the cast of characters in *The House of God* deep into the narrative. The scene occurs in the emergency ward. The two cops are presented as a study in contrasts. The sergeant "is huge, barrel-shaped, with red hair growing out of and into most of the slitty features on his fat red face" (72). Officer Quick is a "matchstick, decked out, facially, in white of skin and black of hair, with vigilant eyes and a large and worrisome mouth filled with many disparate teeth." Both are Irish. Their Irishness is all the more glaring given their work in the predominantly Jewish House of God. It is the sergeant's considered judgment that the Irish and Jews are similar in one significant respect. Humorously, he declares: "In their respect for the family unit, and the concomitant fucked-up nature of their lives" (Shem, *House*, 2003 72).

The favorite line from the two Irish cops is: "Would we be policemen if we were not?" (73). This is their standard response when they exhibit more knowledge about a question or event than is expected. Their extensive knowledge in matters medical is the product of their jabbering with their friends, the interns and residents. When Roy asks where they, as Irish cops, learned about Freud, their response is fabulous: "Where? Why, here, man, here, from spending the last twenty years, here, five nights a week, in trialogues of discussion with fine young overeducated men like you. Better than night school, more broad and useful. And we get paid to attend" (117). Their preferred interlocutor is one they can describe as "a textbook in himself," like the surgeon Gath, and Cohen, the "sophisticated, jocular, and unrestrained resident in psychiatry" (117). When they have an opportunity to jabber with the Fat Man, they are all smiles, "for twenty minutes of Fat Man chat is a gift horse we shall look everywhere but in the mouth" (73).

The two cops are masters of active listening, often offering humorous comebacks grounded in an exquisite understanding of the struggles at the House of God. When Roy is on emergency ward duty, they welcome him by acknowledging his bohemian sexuality, which they understand as a commonplace coping strategy for successive waves of interns: "Welcome to this little bit of Ireland in the heart of the Hebrew House. Your track record for the naughty upstairs ward has preceded you, and we know that you will amuse all of us with stories of passion in the long chill nights to come" (172). The idiosyncrasies of the two cops interacting with those of other members of the House of God become a source of stabilizing humor for Roy. Roy gets to talk to Gilheeny and Quick often when on emergency ward duty. The two cops become veritable textbooks in themselves simply from actively listening to the knowledge of the interns.

Gilheeny and Quick are a reservoir of institutional memory. Their twenty years of work in the emergency ward and steady pumping of information about medicine and life from the bright interns of the House of God endow them with superb diagnostic capacities about what ails the interns. They reciprocate the continuing education they receive from the interns by occasionally serving as dubious mentors for some of the naive interns. For example, they set up a blind date for Grenade Room Dubler. During Dubler's date with Lulu, in the backseat of the officer's police vehicle, a shocked Dubler discovers that Lulu is a transsexual, complete with a hardened male member! The officers regard themselves as educators and textbooks in themselves of a different sort.

There is a twisted element of justice when Roy Basch saves the relationship between Sergeant Gilheeny and Officer Quick, only to be saved himself from a complete mental meltdown by the two cops and others who love him. In a sense, the lives that thrive in the House of God are those that manage to make and maintain healthy connections. The connected can receive care when they need it. There is an episode in the book in which Gilheeny is shot. Roy and his House of God associates do all they can to restore the sergeant to his partner in fighting crime, Officer Quick. The coordinated intervention of police, hospital, and family system snatches Gilheeny from the jaws of death and ensures him sufficient health for many more days of crime fighting. The tables turn when Roy succumbs to the sanity-breaking pressures of his House of God internship. It occurs at the end of the internship. Roy plans to join Berry, his steady romantic partner, for a Marcel Marceau show. Something snaps in his world and he decides to spend the night caring for his patient, Mrs. Pedley. It takes the intervention of Berry, with the help of the two cops and Chuck, to physically remove Roy from the House of God, transport him to the theater, sandwich him and Berry between Gilheeny and Quick, and allow the Marceau show to work its magic. The MVI intern who was almost lost is now found: "As we parted from them Gilheeny, touched, said, 'Good night, friend Roy. We'd been worried that we'd lost you'" (327).

It is ironic that the cops have more insight into caring than the physician supervisors do. Their presence underscores the deficiencies of the supervising physicians and of American medical education. Those not in the system have a greater sense of caring and more effectiveness than the highly esteemed teaching physicians. This underscores the deficits of the training in effective care of patients.

It might be that our world is prone to madness, hence the gravitational pull of psychiatry in *The House of God,* a pull that yields among its candidates the two Irish cops. By the end of the internship year, five have indicated their desire to pursue a residency in psychiatry: the Runt, Chuck, Eddie, the Crow, and the MVI. Everyone is shocked when to these raised hands are added those of Gilheeny and Quick. Of course the two cops cannot become psychiatrists, but thanks to their connections with Grenade Room Dubler, who has become "the bearded President of the Psychoanalytic Institute," they can become lay analysts. Their services would be in demand by the law enforcement establishment, populated on both sides by the warped and criminally perverted, one side more so than the one that wears the respected uniforms.

Zock's Insight

The Zock family is introduced as Roy first approaches the House of God: "I stood in the steamy heat outside a huge urine-colored building which a sign said was THE HOUSE OF GOD. A ball and chain were demolishing one wing, to make way, as a sign said, for THE WING OF ZOCK" (Shem, *House,* 1978 24).

As the story progresses, we learn more about the Zocks, first through their physician:

> Even at the BMS, I'd heard of the Pearl. Once the Chief Resident, he had soon abandoned academics in pursuit of cash, had snatched the beginnings of his own practice from his older partner when the latter was away on a Florida vacation, and with a quick entry into computer technology that fully automated his office, the Pearl had become the richest of the rich House privates. A gastroenterologist with his personal X-Ray machine in his office, he serviced the wealthiest bowels in town. He was the retained physician of the Family of Zock, whose Wing of Zock jackhammers would make us throw our stethoscopes away. Well-groomed, glittering with gems, in a handsome suit, he was a master with people, and in a few seconds he had us in the palm of his hand. (27)

We come to know the Zocks mostly indirectly. They are rich, able to afford and control access, but not necessarily any better off in the end in outcomes of medical care. The building of the Tower of Zock gets in the way of medical care while promising to make it better. We finally encounter Nate Zock late in the work. "There lay Nate, a rubbery-faced sixty, a bit booze-riddled, but with wealth in his manner and in his mien. Even hassled by the herd, he was calm" (383).

After Roy is appropriately directive with the overbearing Zock family, he evaluates Nate Zock. He tells him that a minimal workup is likely to be most helpful and most likely to promote healing. It is clear that Mr. Zock likes Roy's candor and his ability not to be bowed by the "herd" of Zock relatives. In the end, he honors Roy with a dedication in the Wing of Zock.

The Zocks have "special access" due to their money and contributions. This access does not save Old Lady Zock when the needs of another patient draw the staff away from the monitors in the Cardiac Care Unit. Money cannot buy luck. Money cannot control outcomes. There is an inadvertent justice in the work of fate.

CONCLUSION

As noted in the book, cynical humor is commonly used by physicians in training to protest the disrespect, the overwork, the impotence intrinsic to hospital-based care and training. Initially, the protagonist finds that humor preserves sanity from day to day, but failure to address the intrinsic injustices eats away at Roy's soul. The destructive power of the situation is made clear in Potts's death by suicide.

The distributive justice of fairness and of meeting individuals' needs is mostly notable for its absence or violation throughout the narrative. It is the underlying impetus for the need for the aggressive cynical humor. Indeed, it may well be the overwhelming sense of impotence against the many areas of unfairness and injustice that drives the bravado of the surrealistic sex scenes. In Fats, we see that humor and cynicism can camouflage the patient-centered justice at the bedside. By the end, we see that the truth, like the physical examination of the patient, cannot best be revealed in its entirety all at once, but rather through the revelation of parts in an orderly and formalized way. We must be prepared to receive the secrets. We must prove ourselves worthy through the quest of knowledge in medical school and the night journey of internship. Sympathy. *Sym*—together. *Pathos*—suffering, enduring. While it is arguable that unlimited suffering is not a necessary part of the maturing of a physician, there is a special learning intrinsic to this process. Physicians in training need to struggle, suffer, and endure but also need to redirect their energies, not against disease, not against the patient, not against the system, but with the patient for the healing aspect of the connection.

WORKS CITED

Shem, Samuel. *The House of God.* New York: Dell, 1978.
———. *The House of God.* New York: Dell, 2003.

Wearing the Ring of Gyges in the House of God

JULIE M. AULTMAN

The main source of illness in this world is the doctor's own illness: his compulsion to try to cure and his fraudulent belief that he can.

SAMUEL SHEM, THE HOUSE OF GOD

Then virtue is the health and beauty and well-being of the soul, and vice the
disease and weakness and deformity of the same?

PLATO, REPUBLIC

In Plato's *Republic,* Glaucon tells the story of Gyges, a shepherd in the service
of the ruler of Lydia. After a great deluge of rain and an earthquake, the ground
opened and a chasm appeared at the place where he was pasturing. Wander-
ing down this chasm, Gyges found, among other riches, a hollow bronze horse
with little doors containing a corpse within. Gyges pilfered the corpse's only
possession—a gold ring—and placed it on his hand. It was by chance, during an
assembly of shepherds making their monthly report, that Gyges realized the great
power his ring held. When Gyges turned the collet of the ring toward himself,
he became invisible, and when turning it outward, he regained visibility. Having
this newfound power, "he immediately managed things so that he became one
of the messengers who went up to the king, and on coming there he seduced
the king's wife and with her aid set upon the king and slew him and possessed
his kingdom" (Plato 360b).

The moral of this tale, according to Glaucon, is that if there were such a
power available to people, everyone would act the same way as Gyges. Under
normal circumstances, he argues, people do what is ethically right only because
they lack the power to do what they really want. Glaucon's claim, however, lacks
"the reasoning and the language of the opposite party, of those who commend
justice and dispraise injustice" (Plato 362e). In challenging Glaucon's claim,
Plato reveals to Glaucon that being virtuous depends on the value of the virtue
itself, not the rewards and honors a good reputation may bring. Thus, there are
people who do what is ethically right because leading a good life is intrinsically
valuable, regardless of the rewards and honors it brings.

In *The House of God,* within the hierarchy of health care professionals, there is a desire to wear the ring of Gyges, to reap the benefits of injustice, while at the same time maintaining a virtuous reputation. As the narrating character, Dr. Roy Basch, describes, "The House medical hierarchy was a pyramid—a lot at the bottom and one at the top. Given the mentality required to climb it, it was more like an ice-cream cone—you had to lick your way up. From constant application of tongue to next uppermost ass, those few toward the top were all tongue" (Shem 14). Those at the top, the Slurpers, possess great power but at the same time promote injustice within the clinical setting such that cure, the only perceived goal of medicine, takes precedence over both patient *and* physician care. One valuable lesson learned by all who witness the "slurping" is how to recognize this injustice. As lessons such as this one are learned, and relationships between physician and patient, resident and intern, and physician and other are established and nurtured, many of the characters of *The House of God* arguably lead their lives as virtuous individuals, regardless of the unethical acts they may perform or the vice-laden reputations they may carry. In the end, these characters show us the value of virtue within medical practice and how an indispensable, virtuous character can lead to overall good patient care.

In this essay, I critically diagnose the problems associated with virtue theory in the resolution of ethical conflict in medicine but also argue that virtue theory does have a place in medical practice regardless of its limitations. I then illustrate how virtue theory plays a significant role in the moral development of certain characters in *The House of God,* suggesting that a person can lead a virtuous professional life even after having committed immoral or unprofessional acts. Finally, I examine the importance of virtue theory in the moral development of physicians, namely through role modeling, using examples from *The House of God.*

VIRTUE IN MEDICINE

Discussions of virtue likely began in the sixth century B.C. and then appeared in concrete form in approximately 360 B.C. in the *Republic,* where Plato introduced four cardinal, or primary, virtues—wisdom, temperance, courage, and justice—each relating directly or indirectly to the soul (Ferngren and Amundsen 9). The Platonic scheme of the soul involved three parts—the intellect, will, and appetite—to which the virtues of wisdom, courage, and temperance correspond respectively. Justice, the virtue that does not directly correspond to any particular part of the soul, is the virtue that regulates the others. When all the constituent parts of the soul are harmoniously organized and regulated, the best performance of living is achieved. Furthermore, harmony within the soul is analogous to a healthy body, and thus begins the connection between virtues and medicine, where "moral virtue, after the model of human pathology, was regarded not as adherence to an external code or standard, but as a balance of the elements of the soul" (Ferngren and Amundsen 10).

Unlike Plato, Aristotle argued that virtue is not innate, but acquired through the performance of virtuous actions. In training ourselves to be virtuous, according to Aristotle, we need to find balance between the extremes of excess and defect. In what is known as the "doctrine of the mean," Aristotle writes: "Now virtue is concerned with passions and actions, in which excess is a form of failure, and so is defect, while the intermediate is praised and is a form of success; and being praised and being successful are both characteristics of virtue. Therefore virtue is a kind of mean, since, as we have seen, it aims at what is intermediate" (957; bk. 2, ch. 6, par. 1106b).

Since the days of Plato and Aristotle, philosophers and theologians have added to the primary list of moral and nonmoral virtues while emphasizing the significance of virtue theory within moral practice vis-à-vis competing ethical theories such as deontology (duty based) and consequentialism (goal based). For example, contemporary virtue theorist Alasdair MacIntyre understands virtues as dispositions, "which will not only sustain practices and enable us to achieve the goods internal to practices, but which will also sustain us in the relevant kind of quest for the good, by enabling us to overcome the harms, dangers, temptations and distractions which we encounter, and which will furnish us with increasing self-knowledge and increasing knowledge of the good" (211). MacIntyre, in following the Aristotelian tradition, proposes that as dispositions, virtues exhibit three characteristics. First, they are necessary for humans to attain the goods internal to communal practices. Next, virtues sustain communal identities in which individuals can seek the good of their whole lives. And lastly, they sustain traditions that provide practices and individual lives with necessary historical context. These three characteristics suggest that virtue ethics does not focus solely on individuals, but on individuals in relation to their communities; in accordance with the doctrine of the mean, individual good is balanced with the good of community.

Though there are various interpretations as to how the virtues (and which ones) are linked to the culture and practice of medicine, proponents of virtue theory commonly argue that intellectual and moral virtues play a significant role in the lives of practitioners and the institutions and societies they serve. The virtuous physician possesses a moral character and acts accordingly, balancing personal goods with the overall good of his or her institutional, local, and global communities. However, not all moral theorists believe virtues play such a significant role.

Some of the main arguments against virtue theory are based on the perceived difficulty of moral decision making. If two or more virtues are competing, for example, there are no rules or guidelines that suggest one virtue should take precedence over another. Also, there is little explanation as to how virtue leads to morally right actions, especially when the virtues themselves may be interpreted differently among individuals and groups and across cultures.

Though there is no particular systematic method of resolving conflict when there are competing virtues or competing interpretations, some virtue theorists, following an Aristotelian philosophy, would argue that the virtuous individual is able to grasp the unity of the virtues, find balance among them, and determine which action to take even in complex situations. The system of virtues is not free of difficulties and objections, but it is a system that is useful in the medical context, where a virtuous character often shapes and is shaped by the principles and duties an individual follows. In other words, the virtues need not stand alone without further ethical guidance from additional moral theories and principles. So while virtue theory does have its limitations, it plays a significant role in medical ethics and practice along with, for example, duty-based and rule-based ethics.

In *The House of God,* individual characters develop into virtuous physicians, ironically, by finding balance among the vices, challenging and finding meaning in the principles and rules of medical practice, and establishing meaningful relationships with their role models, patients, and others. Finding virtue in the House of God, the hospital affiliated with the BMS (Best Medical School), however, is not an easy task; virtuous characters are hidden beneath unethical acts, unprofessional behavior, and feelings of fear and guilt. In determining which characters possess or acquire virtue, we begin by asking the question, If the characters of *The House of God* were to wear the ring of Gyges, would they do whatever they wanted, and if so, would their actions be motivated by a virtuous character or a character laden with vice?

VICES IN THE HOUSE

Uncovering virtue within *The House of God* requires a careful look at the many vices that may challenge the claim that particular characters are, in fact, virtuous. The more obvious vices include intemperance, callousness, cynicism, self-interest, and dishonesty. Consider first the hedonistic sexual acts between the interns and other members of the health care team.

The culture within *The House of God* challenges most rules of ethics and etiquette, dividing the environment within from the outside world. Illustrating this divide is the legendary sexual encounter between the unattached female nurse and the male doctor in a committed relationship. As the interns acquire some regularity in their clinical responsibilities, they begin to explore the social culture of the House of God, namely the nurses and housekeeping staff housed within. Intern Roy Basch explains, "Without realizing it, perniciously, hand in hand with our growing competence and rising resentment at the way we were being drilled by Jo and the Slurpers, we had begun to, almost without knowing it, as Chuck said, 'get it on' with those erotic ones in the House of God" (Shem 105). Though in a relationship with Berry, Roy has an affair with Molly, a perky nurse who is eager to fulfill all of Roy's sexual desires in every private corner of the House. Roy attempts to cover up this scandalous love affair, feeling too ashamed to tell Berry of his unfaithfulness to her. And though ashamed, he continues to have loveless sex with Molly as a way to escape from the daily realities of being an intern in the House until she realizes Roy is too cynical and destructive for her. Eventually Molly moves on to another intern, Howie Greenspoon, who, according to Roy, was blessed with two traits: "unawareness of self and unawareness of others" (72). Needless to say, Roy is quite surprised to find that Molly is interested in Howie, which causes him to reflect on his infidelity and growing cynicism but does not stop him from having sex with other women, including Selma from social services.

Roy is not alone in his sexual overindulgence, as Chuck, another intern and Roy's best friend, finds erotic pleasure with Hazel, the "Cuban firecracker" from housekeeping (104). And yet Roy and Chuck cannot even compare to Harold "the Runt" Runtsky, an intern first introduced as a short, stocky, shy, and quiet individual who has "trouble standing up to women sexually" (53) but becomes "a four-dimensional sex fiend" (165). The Runt "had moved from two-dimensional magazine sex into a spine tingling sexual adventure with a voracious nurse named Angel" (4). Angel is the Runt's primary object of pleasure and affection; however, he eventually moves on to other women in the House, including a pubescent physical therapist and Rosalie Cohen from social services. In disbelief at the Runt's transformation, Roy and Chuck cannot help but wonder how they created such a sexual deviant.

At one point in *The House of God*, where the line between reality and fantasy blurs, Roy, the Runt, Angel, Molly, and Selma engage in an explicit, drunken orgy of sorts in an on-call room of the House. In providing some justification for these acts of intemperance, Samuel Shem writes, "Sexual activity between female nurse and male doctor figures here as mutual relief, as a refuge for both classes of caregiver from the circumambient illness and death, from everything distasteful and pathetic and futile and repulsive about flesh" (xiv). However, Shem also refers to the sex in the House of God as "sad and sick and cynical and sick . . . for all of us had become deaf to the murmurs of love" (4).

The loveless sex is not the only example of intemperance among the interns. Throughout *The House of God*, the interns continue to drown their fears, sorrows, and frustration in alcohol. Roy explains the reason why Chuck, for example, doesn't go through his internship year without a bottle of Jack Daniels: "Alcohol helped in the House of God, and I think of my best friend, Chuck, the black intern, who was never without a pint of Jack Daniel's in his black bag for those extra-bitter times when he was hurt extra bad by the gomers or the slurping House academics, like the Chief Resident or the Chief of Medicine himself, who were always looking at Chuck as illiterate and underprivileged when in fact he was literate and privileged and a better doc than anyone else in the whole place" (6).

Defined by Plato as a process of doing good, temperance is "almost synonymous with virtue itself, of doing good, of knowing what we know and do not know, of the health of the soul" (Pellegrino and Thomasma 117). For the interns in the House of God, there is little balance between excess and defect when it comes to the bodily pleasures. Arguably, however, the overindulgences of sex and alcohol balance against the defect of life—all the sickness, suffering, despair, and death the interns witness throughout their internship year. Through acts of intemperance the interns seem to believe they are better equipped to care for their sick and dying patients and bear the brunt of criticism from their mentors, who are themselves characters laden with vice when it comes to medical practice.

Instances that cause us to question the presence of virtue within medical practice are the various dehumanizing comments and acts committed by the Slurpers, including Dr. Jo Miller, Dr. Putzel, chief resident Dr. Fishman ("The Fish"), and the chief of medicine, Dr. Leggo. The infamous resident known as the Fat Man, or "Fats," compares these physicians to terrific medical texts lacking in common sense; they only care to know the disease, not the patient, as evidenced by the following excerpt describing Dr. Jo Miller: "They all shared the belief that disease was some wild and hairy monster to be locked up in the neat medical grids of differential diagnosis and treatment. All it took was a little superhuman effort and all would be well. Jo had dedicated her whole life to that effort, and she had little energy for anything else. . . . She needs these patients so badly to fill up the emptiness of her life that she comes in on Sundays and on her nights off" (Shem 91).

While Jo gives the illusion she is a virtuous physician in the House of God, Roy and the other interns realize she is an unethical person merely possessing a virtuous reputation among the other Slurpers. Though intelligent, skillful, committed, and diligent, Jo fails to see beyond the mechanics of medical practice, believing that all patients can and should be cured of their illnesses. As Fats suggests, "Jo should go into research, but she knows that if she did, it would confirm what everybody else knows already—she can't deal with people" (91). Without care and compassion, Jo aggressively treats her patients, even those who have failed her by tragically giving in to their own ill health, such as dear

Dr. Sanders. After Dr. Sanders's death, Jo insists that a postmortem examination should be performed for the sake of science. Having personally cared for Dr. Sanders, Roy tells Jo, "I loved him too much to see his body ripped apart downstairs." In response, Jo exclaims, "That kind of talk has no place in modern medicine," and orders the postmortem against Roy's wishes (159).

One of Jo's obligations is to teach the new interns how to practice *good* medicine; however, what she teaches them is her false belief that all patients need her and everything that ails them should be treated. As patients start out under Jo's care, they become worse. One patient with dementia, Anna O, starts out in "perfect electrolyte balance, with each organ system working as perfectly as an 1878 model could" (90), but as Jo begins to order more and more tests, Anna becomes gravely ill. Finding Roy with Anna one night, Fats asks Roy what he is doing. Roy explains that Jo is going "all-out on her dementia," and he is reluctantly following her orders even though Anna is becoming more ill. Fats's solution for Roy is to do nothing and hide it from Jo—to "continue the workup in purely imaginary terms, BUFF the chart with the imaginary results of the imaginary tests, Anna will recover to her demented state, the workup will show no treatable cause for it, and everybody's happy. Nothing to it." Roy, questioning the ethics behind this deceitful act, is answered by Fats's rhetorical question, "Is it ethical to murder this sweet gomere with your workup?" (91).

So, along with Roy, the interns Chuck and Potts ignore Jo's requests to aggressively treat the gomers, hiding the fact that they are doing nothing by constructing imaginary medical workups with imaginary tests. Though noble in their efforts to save patients from Jo's aggressive treatment, their unethical acts of lying and falsifying medical records seriously call into question the moral goodness of their characters. Yet this is one example of how values may conflict (e.g., honesty conflicting with compassion and beneficence) where the resolution of such a conflict may not rest solely on good intentions or on a person's character, but on particular acts couched in duty and in their consequences. That is, while Roy and the other interns may present themselves as virtuous physicians as they express genuine concern and compassion for their patients, unlike Jo, this alone may not ethically justify the wrongful acts of lying and falsifying medical records. Even though the overall system of health care may be unjust, it would seem that by lying and falsifying records, giving patients treatments they do not need, and omitting treatments they do need, the physicians of the House of God are contributing to this injustice.

Now, it can be argued that Roy and the other interns have little if no choice in deceiving Jo and the other Slurpers as they continue to buff the charts. After all, the Slurpers are in command and most likely would not hear of doing *nothing* for patients. And, as Roy discovers, "BUFF the chart, you automatically BUFF the Slurpers. Not only that, but I soon found out that the more tests I ordered, the more complications there were, the longer the House kept the patients, and the more money the Privates collected" (89–90).

However, by continuing to buff the charts rather than confronting Jo and the others about the abuses of treating the gomers for the sake of self-interest, medical science, and financial gain, the interns desperately cling to the vices of cynicism, injustice, and cowardice, believing nothing is going to change, and they're certainly not the ones to make it happen. In justifying their unethical actions, the interns may believe that the only individuals getting harmed in the process are the gomers, who don't even know they are being harmed. However, they—the interns—are harming themselves as their cynicism, cowardice, and fears consume them.

But are these young interns truly cynical, unjust, and cowardly? And, if so, are they devoid of virtue or just overworked? It is not uncommon for medical students, interns, and residents to develop a cynical attitude over the course of their medical education as they come to the realization that not every patient will go home happy and healthy, and one's own personal health and well-being as a physician may be compromised by sleep deprivation, depression, anxiety, alcohol and substance abuse, and, for some, suicide. For example, when Mrs. Rishenhein, a little old lady in no apparent distress (LOL in NAD), arrests, Roy is surprised to hear himself say, "I wish she would die so I could just go to sleep" (118), then rightfully calls himself an animal for having said such a thing. To make matters worse, Mrs. Rishenhein is one of several patients the Runt is responsible for. Unfortunately, Jo, in charge of the Runt, has made him feel as though he can never do enough, especially when patient after patient keeps dying under his care. Consumed by guilt after being responsible for an endless sea of dying patients and being degraded by Jo, Roy finally tells the Runt to temporarily leave the House. Unfortunately, even away from the House of God, the Runt cannot separate himself from the guilt and his overall lack of confidence. And when Mrs. Rishenhein arrests—another "failure" for the Runt—Roy asks the inebriated Angel to seduce the Runt out of suicide.

The Runt isn't the only intern who cracks in the House of God or who relies on alcohol, sex, and a cynical attitude to get through each day. Overwrought with frustration, anger, and despair in caring for the gomers, and feeling guilty for their unfortunate deaths, two interns, Eat My Dust Eddie and Hyper Hooper, fall apart emotionally and physically. Eat My Dust Eddie takes himself "off the case" of every one of his patients, talking about gomers "only in terms of 'How can I hurt this guy today?' or 'Some of them want us to kill them and some of them don't, and I wish they'd make up their minds 'cause it gets confusing'" (273). When he finally breaks, Drs. Leggo and Fishman decide to give Eddie a rest, thinking he will eventually kill one of the gomers if he continues on in his delusional state of mind. Unfortunately, with Eddie gone, the other interns have to be on call every other night.

Hyper Hooper, working twice as hard, begins "acting like a gomer." Roy reports, "He'd gotten thin, almost scrawny, and neglected his personal hygiene. He began to rock, like a schizophrenic or an old Jew at prayer. . . . The real problem arose when Hooper took to sleeping in the electric gomer beds in restraints, and one day when I came in and found him in an ankle cast and asked him what had happened, he said only GOMERS GO TO GROUND" (276–77). One by one, each of the interns begins to feel the pressures of his internship year, becoming so self-destructive so as to even invite death to replace the unbearable pain.

Intern Wayne Potts is so consumed by guilt for having killed his patient, Lazlow, that he takes his own life. Lazlow, known as the Yellow Man, was diagnosed with fulminant necrotic hepatitis and was under Potts's care. Potts, thinking that he would be able to care for the Yellow Man alone, failed to give him a needed dose of steroids. As Potts continued to care for his other patients, he could not erase the feelings of guilt from his mind. And when the Yellow Man eventually passed away, Potts "had taken the elevator straight to floor eight, had opened a window, and had thrown himself out to his death" (281). Though there may have been a variety of factors contributing to Potts's suicide, such as the recent death of his father, working with the sick and dying, and the incessant nagging from Jo to take better care of his patients, Lazlow's death was the "straw that broke the camel's back." Though it is easy to pity Potts, his suicide reveals a lack of moral courage or fortitude, as he was unable to endure the guilt and overall emotional pain experienced in the House of God. Pellegrino and Thomasma write: "So Aristotle cautions that 'courage is a mean with respect to things that inspire confidence or fear . . . and it chooses or endures things because it is noble to do so, or because it is base not to do so.' So it would be cowardly to escape from poverty or pain by committing suicide, not a virtue of fortitude. Fortitude endures such things" (110).

It would seem as though the lack of temperance, courage, and justice exhibited by the characters in *The House of God* suggests that virtue is an unreachable ideal in medical practice. Overindulgence in sex and alcohol, patient abuse, turfing, buffing, suicide—how could a physician caught up in these vice-laden acts have a virtuous character? In the next section, I show that regardless of the nonvirtuous acts committed in the House of God, the interns develop virtuous characters through the lessons they learn and the role models who teach them that medicine is about becoming skilled not only in the use of technological tools and test ordering but also in developing caring relationships and in acquiring a wholesome professional identity. I also show that no one is completely virtuous, but a virtuous character is achievable through self-reflection. Jo and the other Slurpers, acting without Aristotelian practical wisdom, never understand the gravity of their unbalanced, reward-driven practices of medicine as they continue to ignore the individuals who are suffering most—the patients and their own interns.

VIRTUE FOUND

One way to develop a virtuous character is to recognize, even experience, the vices. While all the characters in *The House of God* seem to lack virtue, we need to delve deeper into who they are and what they have learned from their experiences. Through this exploration we may discover that what lies beneath the surface of these individuals are virtuous characters after all.

Take, for instance, Roy's encounter with a female student who overdoses at a women's college. Unbeknownst to her parents, the student was taken to Man's Best Hospital, a competitor hospital down the road. Roy finds out the student was dead on arrival, but instead of informing the parents of this news, he says to them, "She was taken to the MBH. You'd better go there" (Shem 179). Roy feels guilty about his cowardice and sits, "thinking of the people I'd known who'd been alive and who now were dead, whatever that was" (179). Two astute police officers known as Giheeny and Quick, who have assimilated quite well in the House of God, immediately recognize Roy's guilt. "How hard to deal honestly with death," says Gilheeny. "Harder than the hard elbow of a gomere," says Quick. "And yet that hardness brings out the softness in us all," says the redhead, "the soul in us that makes us cry at births and weddings and wakes and those sad times when the pebbles of the gravedigger dance upon the coffin lid. Sure, and it makes us more human. Yes, this emergency room is not a mean bad place, now, is it?" (180). Roy's failure to disclose the truth—his cowardice—is a result of his inability to deal honestly with death, and perhaps fear of his own mortality when receiving word that someone of such a young age has died. But he *feels* guilty. He acknowledges his cowardice and takes time to reflect on those who have died. He neither makes fun of the situation nor makes a cynical remark; instead, he embraces the moment, confronting who he is as a person. Without this kind of self-reflection, it is difficult for anyone to acquire and maintain virtue. Pellegrino and Thomasma suggest looking at individuals in moral situations before and after in determining whether virtue has been acquired. "The end point," they write, "is a change in human character, a strengthening of virtuous intentions and practices, and a deepening of the disposition to do the morally right thing even when no one is watching" (179).

As Roy continues to care for patients, we see a strengthening of his virtuous intentions and practices. Not too long after he confronts his cowardice, we see him not as the cynical intern, but as the compassionate physician. Roy's compassion is evidenced during an encounter with a twenty-three-year-old married woman who was raped on her way home from a friend's house. She did not go home. She was too ashamed to tell her husband. When she finally makes eye contact with Roy, he takes her in his arms and lets her cry, and he begins crying too. After contacting the patient's husband and performing a rape workup, Roy watches as husband and wife walk out of the hospital. As she pushes away her husband's affectionate arm, Roy can't help but feel "revolted, enraged, pushing the hand away, because the hand can't ever help, because it's a myth that the hand can touch the part that's dead" (222). Regardless of such hopeless thinking, Roy shows genuine empathy; his caring hand *did* touch the part that's dead. Beyond the clinical care and warm embrace, Roy places himself in her shoes, empathetically understanding "her disgust at the ruination of her body by a man" (222).

Lawrence Blum writes, "Compassion involves a sense of shared community/ humanity, of regarding the other as a fellow human being. This means that the other person's suffering (though not necessarily their particular afflicting condition) is seen as the kind of thing that could happen to anyone, including oneself insofar as one is a human being" (319). Roy does not view his twenty-three-year-old patient as "just another patient" or "just another victim of rape." Instead, he regards her as a fellow human being who is suffering in ways similar to his own suffering as his mind and body are metaphorically raped by the Slurpers, the House of God, and his own guilt and fear. But, more significantly, as Roy connects with his patient, he begins to truly understand the meaning of compassion and how even the most compassionate person cannot always completely help the sufferer. Blum writes, "Compassion is not always linked to the prompting of beneficent actions because in many situations it is impossible for the compassionate person to improve the sufferer's condition" (319).

As for Chuck, Eat My Dust Eddie, and the Runt, they each acquire virtue, including the virtues of compassion, prudence, integrity, and fortitude, as they begin to find their purpose within medical practice. Each of them displaces his anger, frustration, and guilt in different destructive ways, whether by drinking, cracking under pressure, or having loveless sex, but in the end, they find solidarity in working together and taking care of each other at their lowest points, while finding the courage to stand up to Jo, the Fish, and the other Slurpers. More specifically, they each show fortitude when they question authority and resist conformity, as they continuously break the rules to benefit their patients and alleviate their own suffering.

Potts, out of all the interns, displays true compassion for all his patients but unfortunately is not able to find balance or an outlet to release his anger, frustration, and guilt. Because Potts cannot find balance, he takes his own life. Potts, however, serves as a reminder to the rest of the interns that in order to succeed—to make it through the trenches of medicine—balance needs to be achieved between a person's personal and professional life, between one's own health and the health of the patient, between the good of the patient and the good of the institution, and, as Aristotle would advise, among such virtues as temperance, compassion, and prudence.

While the interns' experiences in the House of God, along with their solidarity, guide them in developing virtuous characters, their negative and positive role models have even a greater impact on their acquisition of virtue.

ROLE MODELS

Before coming to the self-realization that he is becoming an animal, "a moss brained moose who did not and could not and would not think and talk" (141), Roy tells Berry about the gomers and why Jo, the Fish, and Leggo are making him angry. Berry, in her analysis of Roy's emotions, asserts, "You've got no role models. You don't look up to any of them." When Roy asks, "What about Fats?" Berry responds, "He's sick." "He's not," Roy replies, as he begins to get angry, "Besides there's Chuck and the Runt and Hooper and Eat My Dust. And Potts" (139). But is Fats truly sick or is he a good role model? At the beginning of Roy's internship, Leggo and the Fish reluctantly give Fats the responsibility to orient the new interns to the House of God.

Roy immediately connects with Fats. "I loved him. He was the first person to tell us he knew about our terror" (29). It is Fats who first shows Roy what a gomer is while transitioning him from a BMS student to intern in the House of God. Looking from the outside in, it would seem as though Fats's reference to geriatric patients as gomers is crass and dehumanizing, as suggested by Potts: "Some of us don't feel that way about old people" (29). Making a distinction between dear old people like his own grandmother and gomers, Fats reveals to his interns that "Gomers are human beings who have lost what goes into being human beings. They want to die, and we will not let them. We're cruel to the gomers, by saving them, and they're cruel to us, by fighting tooth and nail against our trying to save them. They hurt us, we hurt them" (29). All the skills and knowledge gained in medical school are questioned by the interns in light of their new role model. On the surface, Fats appears to be a negative role model with his dehumanizing acronyms for patients, blatant disregard for authority, and deceptive medical care as he tells his interns to buff the charts and turf the patients. "The delivery of medical care consisted of a patient coming in and being TURFED out. It was the concept of the revolving door. The problem with the TURF was that the patient might BOUNCE, i.e., get TURFED back. . . . The secret of the professional TURF that did not BOUNCE, said Fats, was the BUFF" (50).

To illustrate the buff to his interns, Fats uses his patient Mr. Rokitansky. Ordering the nurse to get a baseline blood pressure for Mr. Rokitansky, Fats proceeds to put his patient in the Trendelenberg position by adjusting his hospital bed. "In less than thirty seconds Mr. Rokitansky was virtually upside down on his noggin, his feet pointing at forty-five degrees and his head jammed against the headboard, down below the other end" (51). By flipping his patient upside down, Fats is able to raise his blood pressure from 70/40 to 190/100.

> Next Fats showed us how to get just the head of the bed up, for pulmonary edema; the foot of the bed up, for stasis ulcers of the foot; the middle of the bed up, for disorders of the middle. Finally, after he'd done everything with the gomer bed but twist it into a pretzel, using Rokitansky for the holes, he became solemn and said in an excited voice, "I've saved the most important control for last. This button controls the height. Mr. Rokitansky, are you ready?" (51)

With a few more adjustments, Fats teaches his interns how to turf patients to orthopedics (i.e., if a gomer falls, or "goes to ground," and breaks his hip) or to neurosurgery (i.e., if a gomer goes to ground and damages his head). Potts, Chuck, and Roy cannot help but question whether Fats is actually serious or merely trying to cheer up his interns. Nevertheless, Fats clearly disrespects Mr. Rokitansky in the process by using him to demonstrate an unethical way to move patients to other areas of the hospital, transferring their own responsibilities to some other physician.

Such inane and unethical lessons would certainly suggest that Fats is not a positive role model for the interns. Conversely, by the time one finishes reading *The House of God,* it has become clear that the interns uncover the most valuable lessons about what it means to be a good physician, learned primarily from Fats. There are several instances where Fats displays a virtuous character, whether responding to his interns' immoral and wild behaviors or caring for his own patients.

Though buffing the charts and turfing the patients are not exactly acts of honesty, Fats draws the line when Hooper suggests that Fats falsify his patient's consent form for dialysis. After realizing that Hooper falsifies medical posts by placing a pen in unaware or incompetent patients' hands while scribbling their names, Fats yells at Hooper, "Well, stop doing that, it's illegal!" (243). Fats also puts a stop to Roy's cruel and immature joke targeting Dr. Putzel after he "putzels" Roy's discharge for Harry the Horse, a patient who "wills his heart into that crazy rhythm with chest pain" to avoid returning to the nursing home. Roy had a plan to discharge Harry without his knowledge, but Putzel mistakenly told Harry he was going back to the nursing home. Because of Putzel's mistake, Harry was going to remain in the House of God for another six weeks. So, in anger Roy begins a rumor about how some intern has threatened to assassinate Dr. Putzel. "I asked Eddie if he'd heard the rumor about how some tern had threatened to assassinate Putzel, to put a bullet through his brain, and Eddie said, 'Hey high powered medicine! Just what the fucker always deserved!'" (265). Fats, worried that if they continue with these antics, they will never make it through their internship year, tells the interns to lay off Putzel. Though Fats is not necessarily concerned about Putzel's welfare, he is genuinely concerned about his interns' welfare and treats them with as much respect and compassion as he does his patients, with some exceptions, however, as he continues to buff and turf. Jeffrey Burack et al. write that the most important type of modeling "is to treat learners with the compassion and respect with which we want them to treat their patients" (54). Though his methods are nontraditional and controversial, Fats generally treats his interns the way he treats his patients—like human beings. Nevertheless, one may argue that Fats has no compassion or respect for anyone, especially as he contrives various rules that contradict the standard operating procedures of the House of God and most ethical codes and principles.

While Fats appears to be quite evil as he constructs, obeys, and teaches the thirteen laws of *The House of God* (e.g., "Rule #1: Gomers don't die"), there is an undeniable truth to many, if not all, of the laws. And in his search for the truth behind the practice of medicine, Fats arises as a virtuous, and thus positive, role model for his interns. Pellegrino and Thomasma argue that if virtue is not practiced, external rules, such as those dictated by insurance companies, hospital administrators, and pharmaceutical companies, will govern the moral life (178).

Perhaps Fats exemplifies how virtue ought to be understood and practiced in medicine, for he practices his profession honestly and compassionately while disregarding rules and standards that are in the interests of everyone else but the patient. For example, in rule #13, "The delivery of medical care is to do as much nothing as possible," Fats teaches his young interns to care for, but not aggressively treat, the gomers. Fats believes that by aggressively treating rather than caring for this particular patient population, physicians are doing more harm than good. "These people didn't give a damn about their diseases or 'cures'; what they wanted was what anyone wanted: the hand in their hand, the sense that their doctor could care" (Shem 194).

Instead, Fats believes more good can come from treating the gomers like they are "still part of life, part of some grand nutty scheme instead of alone with their diseases, which, most of the time and especially in the clinic, hardly exist at all. With me, they feel they're still part of the human race" (192). Pellegrino and Thomasma write, "In residency training the contact with faculty models is very close, so that the temptation and pressure to conform are difficult to resist. Moreover, in residency, one has chosen a field with which one identifies. To 'rock the boat' by not conforming even to distorted moral values is to alienate oneself and imperil one's career" (181). Even though Fats teaches his interns to buff the charts, turf the patients, and disregard several of the rules and recommendations of the Slurpers—all unethical or unprofessional acts—what the interns learn is that rocking the boat and resisting conformity are often necessary for the overall good of medicine (i.e., the patient's health as well as their own health).

Though many of his actions are ethically controversial, Fats's true character is that of a compassionate and honest physician. His virtuous character does not go unnoticed by the interns when, for example, he informs a patient that she has metastatic cancer—a diagnosis that her own doctor, Dr. Putzel, will never disclose to her. From a corridor Roy watches the interaction between Fats and the patient. "When [Fats] spoke, her eyes pooled with tears. I saw the Fat Man's hand reach out and, motherly, envelop hers. I couldn't watch. Despairingly, I went to bed" (248). By witnessing such interactions between clinician and patient, Roy and the other interns learn the true values of compassion and respect. As Burack et al. write, "The conventional wisdom has remained that values are passively 'caught' rather than actively 'taught': that senior students and trainees emulate the values modeled by senior clinicians, and that such attributes are best taught by demonstration and example in clinical contexts" (49).

In the end, what Fats teaches his interns is to resist conformity, to search beyond the immediate goals of patient care, especially those governed by external forces (e.g., hospital administration, pharmaceutical interest), and that without self-respect, one develops an ill character devoid of virtue. The interns, especially Roy, gain a better understanding of what it means to be a good doctor from Fats, and the type of doctor *not* to become from Jo, Putzel, and the other Slurpers—the negative role models.

Fats, though the most influential role model, is not the only one who teaches the interns what it means to be a good doctor. Regardless of Potts's suicide, he becomes a tragic role model for the other interns, especially for Roy, who finds himself thinking of Potts as a tragic figure, "a guy who'd been a happy towheaded kid you'd love to take fishing with you, who'd mistakenly invested in academic medicine when he'd have been happy in his family business, and who'd become a splattered mess on the parking lot of a hospital in a city he'd despised" (281). Realizing such physically and psychologically damaging effects of medical training, the interns became more reflective in caring for their patients and themselves, taking notice of their vice-laden acts and cynical attitudes.

In addition to the guiding role models who contribute to the interns' moral education, there are various intern-patient relationships in *The House of God* that reveal how much *patients* contribute to the moral development of physicians. One particular instance is the heartfelt relationship between Roy and Dr. Sanders. Roy explains, "We were friends. He was dying with a calm strength as if his dying were part of his life. I was beginning to love him. I began avoiding going into his room" (156). Dr. Sanders was the first patient Roy loved, and who died with uncontrollable suffering. With his head on Roy's lap, helpless and in pain, Dr. Sanders taught Roy invaluable lessons about life, death, and the true meaning of medicine—how to *be* with a patient. Before dying, Dr. Sanders explains to Roy, "I went through the same cynicism—all that training, and then this helplessness. And yet, in spite of all our doubt, we can give something. Not cure, no. What sustains us is when we find a way to be compassionate, to love. And the most loving thing we do is to be with a patient, like you are being with me" (156).

The House of God is a significant text for critically looking at virtue in medicine; it presents us with the realities of virtue theory through the experiences of Fats, Roy, Chuck, Potts, Jo, and the other interns and Slurpers. Samuel Shem teaches us that the virtuous physician is not someone who always follows the rules of ethics and etiquette, but someone who learns the intrinsic value of compassion, respect, integrity, fortitude, and justice, among other virtues, by finding balance between excess and defect through experience and from those who exhibit virtue. By always following the rules, fulfilling explicitly stated duties, a person may not gain a true understanding of virtue and what it means to lead an intrinsically valuable life. Or, as illustrated by Jo's unwillingness to see medicine as something more than a science, her rule following results in an inability to care for her patients as people instead of biological artifacts. Fats, however, makes his own rules based on a deeper understanding of the goals of medicine and what it means to be a virtuous physician. Critical in the interns' development as virtuous physicians are both forms of role models: negative and positive.

MEDICINE AS THE RING OF GYGES

In connecting virtues specifically to the community and practice of medicine, Pellegrino and Thomasma claim there are three important elements of medicine—the nature of illness, the nonproprietary character of medical knowledge, and the oath of fidelity to the patient's interests—which "generate a strong moral bond and a collective responsibility" (36). To uphold this moral bond, physicians should maintain those values that characterize the practice of medicine and define what it is to be a good physician. That is, it is the virtuous physician who is "habitually disposed to act in the patient's good, to place that good in ordinary instances above his own, that he can reliably be expected to do so" (244).

In *The House of God,* those who possess virtuous characters understand the true meaning of medicine beyond the nature of illness and clinical knowledge and skill. Those virtuous characters understand medicine as a special dialogical relationship between patient and physician created through a shared understanding and common reachable goal to alleviate suffering (even if it means having to forgo cure with technology and treatment). The virtuous also understand that medicine is part of their identity, and that without taking care of themselves, alleviating their own suffering, they will not be able to care effectively for the patients they serve.

It is clear from the experiences of Fats, Roy, Chuck, the Runt, Jo, and the other characters within the House of God that medicine has a powerful effect in shaping and defining moral and professional characters. Medicine *is* the ring of Gyges, where those who learn, practice, and identify themselves with medicine have great, unimaginable power. Upon gaining a sense of the nature of their power, the virtuous will not abuse it, while the nonvirtuous, like Gyges, will use it out of self-interest, obtaining only rewards and honors for themselves, as they, in Shem's words, "slurp their way to the top." All the characters wears the ring of Gyges, testing its power and submitting themselves to the vices of intemperance, cowardice, injustice, callousness, cynicism, and dishonesty, among others. However, unlike many of the characters in *The House of God,* Fats along with Roy, Chuck, the Runt, Hooper, and Eddie rise above the vices, gaining a clearer understanding of themselves and the intrinsic value medicine holds when it is not abused.

WORKS CITED

Aristotle. "Ethica Nicomachea (Nicomachean Ethics)." *The Basic Works of Aristotle.* Ed. R. McKeon. New York: Random House, 1941. 935–1126.

Blum, Lawrence. "Compassion." *Morality and the Professional Life: Values at Work.* Eds. Cynthia Brincat and Victoria Wike. Upper Saddle River, NJ: Prentice-Hall, 2000.

Burack, Jeffrey, David M. Irby, et al. "Teaching Compassion and Respect: Attending Physicians' Responses to Problematic Behaviors." *Journal of General Internal Medicine* 14 (1999): 49–55.

MacIntyre, Alasdaire. *After Virtue.* 2nd ed. Notre Dame, IN: Notre Dame University Press, 1984.

Pellegrino, Edmund, D., and David C. Thomasma. *The Virtues in Medical Practice.* New York: Oxford University Press, 1993.

Plato. *The Republic. The Collected Dialogues of Plato.* Ed. E. Hamilton and H. Cairns. Princeton, NJ: Princeton University Press, 1961. 575–844.

Shem, Samuel. *The House of God.* New York: Dell, 2003.

The Laws of the House of God Revisited: or, Sneaking Primary Care into Man's Greatest Hospital

HOWARD BRODY

"What we're saying is that the real problem this year hasn't been the gomers, it's been that we didn't have anyone to look up to."

"No one? No one in the whole House of God?"

"For me," I said, "only the Fat Man."

"Him? He's as kooky as Dubler! You can't mean that, no."

"What we mean, man," said Chuck forcefully, "is this: how can we care for patients if'n nobody cares for us?" (Shem 400)

In this scene, the interns' final confrontation with the Leggo, the chief of the medicine service, at year's end, Chuck gets to voice the moral of the novel, if such can be compressed into one phrase. Roy Basch, the protagonist, makes the point that if the novel has a hero, it is the resident, the Fat Man.

The Leggo protests—the Fat Man cannot be an exemplary physician. He does not fit the mold of the world the chief understands, that of the Slurpers, the academic yes-men who are trying to claw their way to the top, hoping eventually to take over the Leggo's job. The Slurpers care about facts and about diseases. They do not care about patients, and they do not care about the human beings they trample on in their quest for power. The Fat Man has shown the interns that he cares about them; and in his own "kooky" way, he has shown them how to care for the patients too. "More than anyone else, he knew how to be with patients, how to be with us," recalls Basch (409).

If the internship year—today what we'd call the first year of residency—in the House of God is the Inferno and Basch is Dante, then the Fat Man is Virgil. Like Virgil, the Fat Man can show Basch how to make it through the House of God and leave in one piece at the end but cannot accompany him out. All through the novel the Fat Man talks about his future goal—the "bowel run of the stars," the "big fortoona," a practice as a gastroenterologist to Hollywood's rich and famous. But in the last glimpse we catch of him, the Fat Man is standing in the on-call room, indoctrinating the next class of new interns. He seems destined to become the perpetual resident.

One of the ways in which the Fat Man guides Basch and his fellow interns through the inferno of the House of God is by teaching them the laws. Toward the end of the year, Basch shows that he has become a worthy disciple by inventing some of his own laws to add to the list: "Without thinking . . . as if from somewhere else than me . . . I heard myself create a new LAW" (142).

To most readers, the laws of the House of God are simply part and parcel of the novel's comic parody of medicine and internship. They illustrate what in other contexts has been called the "hidden curriculum"—the lessons that the experience of making one's way through medical education teaches the students and residents, even if these lessons form no part of the formal curriculum and even run contrary to the official curricular objectives (Hafferty and Franks 861).

In the usual medical education setting, the hidden curriculum remains implicit and so never openly challenges the hegemony of the formal curriculum. If trainees act weirdly because they are following the dictates of the hidden rather than formal curriculum, those in power can always blame the trainees themselves for their immaturity or recalcitrance. The Fat Man scandalizes the Leggo and the Slurpers because he dares to make the hidden curriculum explicit by proclaiming its laws. No doubt the senior academic physicians who were outraged by *The House of God* when it first appeared, and who rushed to condemn it in print, felt likewise.

Taking the satire of the novel down to a deeper layer of analysis, one might note that senior physicians train their juniors, in many instances, through "clinical pearls." These "pearls" are pithy summaries of clinical wisdom that provide helpful guidance in difficult cases. Kathryn Montgomery, in her study of *How Doctors Think,* observes that the pearls are rough rules of thumb—true for the most part and in general, rather than absolutely—and indeed that there are often contradictory pearls that could be organized in pairs. The pearls therefore stand in opposition to the oft-repeated avowal that medicine is or should be a "science." The pearls are too uncertain and particularistic to function as scientific theories or laws.

Therefore, the laws of the House of God are a sort of double parody of the senior physicians' way of teaching. First, they take the same form as the clinical pearls frequently thrown about by the attendings, even though their content is directly opposed to what those attendings teach and represent. Second, the laws are presented to us *as* laws—that is, as rising to a much higher level of certainty than the attendings' clinical pearls. It is as if the Fat Man has said, "If you want to drive yourself insane all year and also abuse your patients, then listen to what those twits have to say. If you want to survive your internship and allow as many of your patients as possible to survive it too, then you *must* do it the way I tell you." The laws, in short, are a set of anti-pearls (Montgomery 113).

The author of *The House of God* seems to have been rather fond of the laws, compiling them in a list at the conclusion of the text. In roughly a quarter-century of medical practice following my own house staff experience, during which I first read the novel, I have found myself frequently recalling several of these laws, as if they had more to teach about medicine than may first have been evident.

We can, therefore, do much worse in celebration of the novel's anniversary than revisit the laws of the House of God and ask how well they stack up as clinical pearls, as brief lessons that capture critical points about medical practice.

In reviewing the laws, I propose to omit some of them whose purpose seems frankly and solely comic (or pathetic). I will, therefore, have nothing more to say about laws VIII, IX, XI, and XII.

I. GOMERS DON'T DIE.

The novel's glossary defines a gomer, short for "Get out of my emergency room," as "a human being who has lost—often through age—what goes into being a human being" (424). The notion that a demented elderly person is somehow no longer human is a frequently expressed sentiment of residents, who may be of an age that makes it difficult to empathize with the elderly and can only see how much work goes into their medical treatment. Today we can no longer afford to look aside as others employ such dehumanizing language. To keep with the spirit of the novel, however, I will retain the original phrase.

The Fat Man explains this law:

> "This is too sad. He's going to die."
> "No, he's not," said Fats. "He wants to, but he won't." . . .
> "That's ridiculous. Of course they die."
> "I've never seen it, in a whole year here," said Fats.
> "They have to."
> "They don't. They go on and on. Young people—like you and me—die, but not the gomers. Never seen it. Not once."
> "Why not?"
> "I don't know. Nobody knows. It's amazing. Maybe they get past it. It's pitiful. The worst." (43–44)

While it is tempting to dismiss this entire passage as an unacceptable dehumanization of the elderly or mentally impaired, I would submit that there are a few insights that ought not be thrown away with the bath water. For one thing, it is certainly not the case that the typical first-year resident will never see an elderly demented patient die. But it is the case that the resident will usually also see a number of younger people die, and these deaths will probably take a greater emotional toll and be remembered far longer. The deaths of younger people, in our scheme of the world, seem as if they should have been preventable and haunt the physician longer as imagined personal failures. And the young resident can more readily identify with the younger patient and so especially be haunted by this glimpse of his or her own mortality.

It is also the case, as the SUPPORT study has shown us, that despite several decades of bioethicists and others preaching about quality of life and death with dignity, the modern hospital can all too often be an institution that thwarts our best efforts to stop aggressive life-prolonging treatment, even after it can do no good and after the patient and family have made clear that they do not wish it. When the institution proceeds to inflict this suffering and indignity on the elderly dying patient, it is often the house staff and the nurses who are made to be the tools of the institution's cruelty and who therefore suffer the greatest moral distress.

The house staff and nurses feel badly about causing suffering among the elderly and terminally ill because they have been seduced into following the law proposed by the Leggo—"Physicians should always do everything for every patient forever" (Montgomery 257). We will see that the Fat Man's final law, Law XIII, is the direct antithesis of this.

II. GOMERS GO TO GROUND.

The Fat Man cites this law when he writes an order to place a football helmet on Ina, a demented elderly patient. No matter how securely restrained, he says, these patients always manage to get out of their restraints and fall out of bed. In this practice, the Fat Man shows himself to be remarkably prescient, at least in ordering the protective gear. In hindsight, he realizes that he erred, because he allowed the interns to write orders for the restraints, "leaving her tied down six ways from Sunday" (46).

It has taken the geriatricians all these years to convince us that physical restraints don't work, when it takes us five minutes to put them on and the patient has twenty-four hours per day to figure out how to escape them. Instead what happens all too often is that restraints kill patients through strangulation or other equally gruesome means. We are finally learning that we need more humane environmental modification to prevent injury from falls among the elderly. We need Fats's football helmet, or placement of patients' mattresses on the floor, or, even better, more intensive nursing supervision.[1]

III. AT A CARDIAC ARREST, THE FIRST PROCEDURE IS TO TAKE YOUR OWN PULSE.

A patient walks into the hospital. He is clearly not a gomer—he's relatively young, talks coherently, is likeable. The next minute he turns blue and slumps to the floor. The shocked interns freeze like deer caught in headlights. The Fat Man, who till then has been coolly reading the stock reports in the newspaper, leaps up and smoothly and competently runs the code that restores the patient to life. On his way back to the newspaper, he reminds the interns of this law.

In much of medicine, one does damage by doing too much too quickly (Law XIII). There are a few times in medicine where one harms the patient by not doing the right thing quickly enough. In these latter instances, the physician's natural sense of panic is his or her worst enemy. Taking a second or two to slow down—taking one's own pulse virtually if not actually—is wise advice.

It might seem that worrying about one's own pulse in an emergency is self-indulgent. George Engel reminded us that the person of the physician is, or should be, a finely tuned scientific instrument (Engel). The physician takes a medical history and does a physical examination—in short, observes the patient—and thereby provides the basic data from which all further medical reasoning springs. Taking a moment to calibrate that instrument before any encounter, but especially in an emergency, is prudent (Novack, Suchman, et al.). It allows the physician to be there fully with and for the patient.

IV. THE PATIENT IS THE ONE WITH THE DISEASE.

Most of the laws, at first hearing, sound callous. This law at first seems to justify emotional detachment and lack of empathy.[2] By contrast, Charon reads it in a positive way, as a statement that "one wants to diminish one's own private concerns toward giving pride of place to the patient's concerns" (133).

A middle-ground reading is that Law IV calls for setting the emotional distance between physician and patient at just the right place along the spectrum between cold detachment and overidentification, or enmeshment. Montgomery humanizes the right sort of detachment for us as follows: "After all, how to be attentive to another human being without losing oneself is a problem every human being struggles with in one way or another: how to care for children, spouse, parents, friends without being overwhelmed. (And if we do not struggle, it may be because we have reinforced ourselves with something like the clinician's detachment.)" (173).

The Fat Man provides this law for the interns when the Slurpers try to use the interns' natural mistakes to demoralize and dehumanize them. Don't repeat your mistakes, he tells them. But if your patients are suffering, don't take that suffering home with you like an albatross hung around your neck. Don't let guilt make you imagine that you are the one who's sick.

Patients want their physicians to empathize with them and also to be strong. When patients feel weak in the face of their illnesses, they can take heart in the physician's fortitude—she has been there before and seen this threat, and she knows nevertheless that the patient can prevail. The physician with empathy wants to know how the experience of illness is affecting the patient, how the patient is bearing up. When the physician starts to imagine that he has the disease, that he is suffering more than the patient, the opportunity for support and fortitude is lost. Overidentification with the patient's suffering is a kind of self-absorption that robs the patient of the strength he has a right to expect from his doctor.

V. PLACEMENT COMES FIRST.

This law arises from the fear that the gomer transferred from a nursing home will be treated for several days in the hospital and recover, only for the intern to discover that the nursing home has sold that patient's bed in the meantime, condemning the patient (and the intern) to a prolonged hospitalization until another bed can be found. Stated in its bald form, this law is as insensitive as all the others, suggesting that even before one has diagnosed or treated the disease, one should be thinking of the most expeditious way to get rid of the patient.

Yet no patient comes to the hospital with the intent of moving in and living there. The law makes a lot of sense if it is altered slightly: "Early on in the hospital stay, be sure to identify the end goals of hospitalization, what outcome is being sought for the patient, and how one will know that the endpoint has been reached."

In many years of doing hospital ethics consultation on internal medicine wards or in intensive care units, I identified a syndrome that I called "the case of the missing plans." The team of caregivers would be split over the management of the patient, often whether or not to write a do-not-resuscitate order. Inspecting the chart, I would find, each day, a full set of plans to address whatever had been out of whack during the morning when rounds were made—tests to look for infection, a change in dose of insulin to better manage blood sugar, and so on. But nowhere would I find any statement of the long-term plans for the hospitalization, the goals that were supposed to be met for the patient's care overall. When I would ask the team what these plans were, the first reaction would be blank stares. As soon as I could get the team engaged in addressing the plans and goals for the entire hospital stay, whatever the supposed ethical problem I had been called to consult on immediately vanished.

VI. THERE IS NO BODY CAVITY THAT CANNOT BE REACHED WITH A NUMBER FOURTEEN NEEDLE AND A GOOD STRONG ARM.

The Fat Man's take on this law is highly questionable: "You learn on the gomers, so that when some young person comes into the House of God dying . . . you know what to do, you do good, and you save them" (89). In Fats's defense, it should be said that if he had his way, the treatment of the gomers would follow Law XIII, "The delivery of medical care is to do as much nothing as possible." But the Slurpers higher up the ladder will not allow this sensible approach and, in pursuit of academic ideals, keep demanding that each patient be worked up for dozens of rare diseases they do not have, and for which the workup process would kill them much sooner than the disease would. So let us not condemn Fats if he decides that the only way for the interns to survive in this inferno is to try not to kill the elderly demented patients but also to use them as teaching fodder.

Still, I would argue that this law is best observed in the breach. This law typifies the machismo of the successful house officer of the era when *The House of God* was written. Once you have learned that you can invade any bodily space with a long enough needle, the question remains—why should you? When a life can be saved, it is good to have the skills. When no good can be served, when it is really a matter of showing off, the fearsome needle ought to remain sheathed. Most of the time, Law XIII takes priority over Law VI.

VII. AGE + BUN = LASIX DOSE

Lasix (furosemide) is a powerful diuretic that was fairly new on the scene when the novel was written. When the kidney is not making urine as it ought, one marker of the dysfunction is an increase in the blood urea nitrogen, which can be measured by a laboratory test commonly called BUN. As patients get older, their kidneys usually decline in function.

A patient with healthy kidneys, given a low dose of furosemide, will spend an inordinate amount of the remainder of that day in the vicinity of bathrooms. As the kidneys become less and less healthy, or as the patient has become used to routinely receiving higher doses of furosemide, even large doses will do little. Yet if one finally gives a really whopping dose, the kidneys will usually respond. And if the patient has congestive heart failure—one of the most common conditions that land an older patient in the hospital—the diuresis prompted by the furosemide could be lifesaving.

Law VII draws laughs from medical trainees because it stands in stark contrast to the elegant and complicated formulas for determining the doses of medicines that fill popular "peripheral brains"—in *The House of God* days, spiral-bound pocket volumes such as the *Washington Manual of Medical Therapeutics;* today, programs loaded onto PDAs. But, as the Fat Man insists, the law does work as a rough guide to force the inexperienced house officer to use a dose of the medication that would otherwise look scary.

Law VII, like Law VI, must be taken in conjunction with Law XIII. One can, in macho fashion, chemically flog a dying kidney to force it to release a bit of urine. In the fluid overload that marks congestive heart failure, this can be beneficial. But one always has to ask, Does making the kidney produce urine do anything to improve the overall outlook of the patient? Or is it one more example of "doing something" that makes us feel good, and our patients feel worse?

X. IF YOU DON'T TAKE A TEMPERATURE, YOU CAN'T FIND A FEVER.

This law, one of Basch's own inventions, sets the stage for Law XIII. One way of assisting patients to recover by "doing as much nothing as possible" is to forgo useless diagnostic testing.

There are two major ways that much of the testing done by house staff in hospitals can be useless. One is testing for which a positive answer would still not alter the patient's treatment plan. The other is testing for which a positive result is much more likely statistically to be a false rather than a true positive, which leads to much more invasive testing before its falsity can be established (Mathers and Hodgkin).

XIII. THE DELIVERY OF MEDICAL CARE IS TO DO AS MUCH NOTHING AS POSSIBLE.

The specialty of family practice has been labeled an American medical counter-culture (Stephens). My own fondness for Law XIII can probably be traced directly to my training in family practice, as we called it then (now "family medicine" is preferred). At various points in my family practice training, I was told that my specialty had two laws of its own. One is Sutton's law: "Go where the money is." No, family physicians don't get rich. Proper translation: "Spend the most time and energy looking for the most probable diagnoses, since in the unselected population you are going to be seeing daily, these are by far the most common. Spend very limited time and energy looking for rare diagnoses." The other useful law for family practice is Landers's law: "If it ain't broke, don't fix it." Both tie in very nicely with Law XIII. No wonder the Slurpers and the Leggo were scandalized by the Fat Man; he was a family physician, undercover, invading their bastion of academic internal medicine.

Amateur medical historians are fond of saying that even though medicine goes back much further than the Ebers papyrus and Hippocrates, it was only around the start of the twentieth century that the likelihood that a visit to the doctor would improve your health started to exceed the chances that you would become worse. How was it that the human race did not become extinct during all those millennia when medicine had so little to offer? It must be because the human body is extremely adept at self-correction and self-healing. Successful medicine is something like martial arts—one should seek to go with that flow of energy rather than to oppose it.

Once one has excluded immediately life-threatening conditions, doing nothing can accomplish at least two useful things. First, and most obviously, the condition may resolve spontaneously. Second, the condition may evolve in a direction by which the underlying disease can more obviously declare itself. At that later but still treatable stage, the disease can be diagnosed with a rifle workup, whereas earlier, if one had made the diagnosis at all, it could only have come from an expensive and confusing shotgun workup.

"Doing nothing" must be carefully qualified. The world of the House of God cares only for physiological measurements and discounts human contact and relationships. The good family physician or other primary care specialist "does nothing" only in the House of God sense. In the more comprehensive sense, she does a great deal. She reassures, she cajoles, she promises regular attendance and surveillance. "I am with you throughout the entire course of this illness, whatever it turns out to be," she promises. "And then I will still be with you after it resolves." That promise, that presence, as much as knowing facts from textbooks, is the essence of doctoring. It is "doing something" with a vengeance.

At the end of the year, Basch thanks the Fat Man: "You showed me that a guy can stay in medicine and still be himself, that besides the Leggo and [the Slurpers], there's another way" (372). For Basch, the only way at the end of the inferno year that he could stay in medicine and still be himself was to go into psychiatry. Actually, the Fat Man had shown him that he had a career cut out for him in primary care medicine, which is as close as one can get to psychiatry while still taking care of patients' physical complaints as well. But in the world of the House of God, leaving an internal medicine residency to go into psychiatry was as much heresy as could be tolerated; seeking a career as a primary care physician was way too far over the edge.

CONCLUSION

The House of God is a satirical novel that works largely via irony. One of the novel's major ironies is that the laws of the House of God, at first glance little more than inarticulate screams of revenge from the house staff toward those who are abusing and dehumanizing them, actually contain a great deal of medical wisdom. Indeed, they contain greater wisdom about the management of sick human beings than the academic internal medicine approach in which the House prided itself on teaching its interns and residents. Thirty years later, they are still worthy of careful review.

NOTES

1. For an example of geriatric research documenting the lack of benefits with, and the dangers of, physical restraints, see Capezuti et al.

2. This reading is suggested by one astute observer of medical education, Frederic Hafferty (31).

WORKS CITED

Capezuti, E., L. Evans, N. Strumpf, and G. Maislin. "Physical Restraint Use and Falls in Nursing Home Residents." *Journal of the American Geriatrics Society* 44 (1996): 627–33.

Charon, Rita. *Narrative Medicine: Honoring the Stories of Illness.* New York: Oxford University Press, 2006.

Engel, George L. "How Long Must Medicine's Science Be Bound by a Seventeenth Century World View?" *The Task of Medicine: Dialogue at Wickenberg.* Ed. Kerr L. White. Menlo Park, CA: Kaiser Family Foundation, 1988. 113–36.

Hafferty, Frederic W. "In Search of a Lost Cord: Professionalism and Medical Education's Hidden Curriculum." *Educating for Professionalism: Creating a Culture of Humanism in Medical Education.* Ed. Delese Wear and Janet Bickel. Iowa City: University of Iowa Press, 2000. 11–34.

Hafferty, Frederic W., and Ronald Franks. "The Hidden Curriculum, Ethics Teaching, and the Structure of Medical Education." *Academic Medicine* 9 (1994): 861–71.

Mathers, N., and P. Hodgkin. "The Gatekeeper and the Wizard: A Fairy Tale." *British Medical Journal* 298 (1989): 172–74.

Montgomery, Kathryn. *How Doctors Think: Clinical Judgment and the Practice of Medicine.* New York: Oxford University Press, 2006.

Novack, D. H., A. L. Suchman, et al. "Calibrating the Physician: Personal Awareness and Effective Patient Care." *Journal of the American Medical Association* 278 (1997): 502–9.

Shem, Samuel. *The House of God.* New York: Dell, 1978.

Stephens, G. G. "Family Medicine as Counter-Culture." *Family Medicine* 21 (1989): 103–9.

The SUPPORT Principal Investigators. "A Controlled Trial to Improve Care for Seriously Ill Hospitalized Patients." *Journal of the American Medical Association* 274.20 (Nov. 22, 1995): 1591–98.

Literary Perspectives
and Criticism

Mayhem at the Hospital

JOHN UPDIKE

We expect the world of doctors. Out of our own need, we revere them; we imagine that their training and expertise and saintly dedication have purged them of all the uncertainty, trepidation, and disgust that we would feel in their position, seeing what they see and being asked to cure it. Blood and vomit and pus do not revolt them; senility and dementia have no terrors; it does not alarm them to plunge into the slippery tangle of the interior organs, or to handle the infected and the contagious. For them, the flesh and its diseases have been abstracted, rendered coolly diagrammatic and quickly subject to infallible diagnosis and effective treatment. *The House of God* is a book to relieve you of these illusions; it does for medical training what *Catch-22* did for the military life—displays it as farce, a melee of blunderers laboring to murky purpose under corrupt and platitudinous superiors. In a sense *The House of God* is more outrageous than *Catch-22,* since the military has long attracted (indeed, has forcibly drafted) detractors and satirists whereas medical practitioners as represented in fiction are generally benign, often heroic, and at worst of drolly dubious efficacy, like the enthusiastic magus, Hofrat Behrens, of Thomas Mann's *The Magic Mountain.*

Not that the young interns and residents and nurses conjured up by Samuel Shem are not sympathetic; they all bring to the grisly funhouse of hospital care a residue of their initial dedication, and the most cynical of them, the Fat Man, is the most effective and expert. Our hero, Roy Basch, is possessed of a buoyant innocence and a persistent—for all the running hypochondria of his hectic confessional narrative—health. Three windows look out of the claustral hospital onto the sunlit lost landscape of happiness: sex, boyhood nostalgia, and basketball. The sex is most conspicuous, and in the orgies with Angel and Molly acquires an epic size and pornographic ideality. A glimpse of Molly's underpants becomes, in one of the book's many impetuous parlays of imagery, a sail bulging with the breath of life:

> . . . in the instant between the sit down, there's a flash of the fantasy triangle, the French panty bulging out over the downy *mons* like a spinnaker before the soft blond and hairy trade winds. Even though, medically, I knew all about these

organs, and had my hands in diseased ones all the time, still, knowing, I wanted it and since it was imagined and healthy and young and fresh and blond and downy soft and pungent, I wanted it all the more.

In the prevailingly morbid milieu, spurts of lust arrive from a world as remote as the world of Basch's father's letters, with their serenely illogical conjunctions. Sexual activity between female nurses and male doctors figures here as mutual relief, as a refuge for both classes of caregiver from the circumambient illness and death, from everything distasteful and pathetic and futile and repulsive about the flesh. It is the co-ed version of the groggy camaraderie of the novice interns: "We were sharing something big and murderous and grand."

The heroic note, not struck as often or blatantly as the note of mockery, is nevertheless sounded, and is perhaps as valuable to the thousands of interns who have put themselves to school with the pedagogic elements of Shem's distinctly didactic novel: the thirteen laws laid down by the Fat Man; the doctrines of gomer* immortality and curative minimalism; the hospital politics of TURFING and BUFFING and WALLS and SIEVES; the psychoanalysis of unsound doctors like Jo and Potts; the barrage of medical incidents that amounts to a pageant of dos and don'ts. It would be a rare case, I imagine, that a medical intern would encounter and not find foreshadowed somewhere in this *Gray's Anatomy* of dire possibilities.

Useful even to its mostly straight-faced glossary, *The House of God* yet glows with the celebratory essence of a real novel, defined by Henry James as "an impression of life." Sentences leap out with a supercharged vitality, as first-novelist Shem grabs the wheel of that old hot-rod, the English language:

The jackhammers of the Wing of Zock had been wiggling my ossicles for twelve hours.

From the ruffled front unbuttoned down past her clavicular notch showing her cleavage, to her full tightly held breasts, from the red of her nail polish and lipstick to the blue of her lids and the black of her lashes and even to the twinkly gold of the little cross from her Catholic nursing school, she was a rainbow in a waterfall.

We felt sad that someone our age who'd been playing ball with his six-year-old son on one of the super twilights of summer was now a vegetable with a head full of blood, about to have his skull cracked by the surgeons.

---

*A far-gone, usually elderly patient, from the acronym GOMER: Get Out of My Emergency.

We have here thirty-year-old Roy Basch's belated *Bildungsroman,* the tale of his venture into the valley of death and the truth of the flesh, ending with his safe return to his eminently sane and sanely sensual Berry. Richard Nixon—the most fascinating of twentieth-century Presidents, at least to fiction writers— and the mounting Watergate scandal form the historical background of the novel, pinning it to 1973–74. *The House of God* could probably not be written now, at least so unabashedly; its lavish use of freewheeling, multi-ethnic cari- cature would be inhibited by the current terms "racist," "sexist," and "ageist." Its Seventies sex is not "safe"; AIDS does not figure among the plethora of vividly described diseases; and a whole array of organ transplants has come along to enrich the surgeon's armory. Yet the book's concerns are more timely than ever, as the American health-care system approaches crisis condition—ever more overused, overworked, expensive, and beset by bad publicity, as grotesqueries of mismanagement and fatal mistreatment outdo fiction in the daily newspapers. As it enters its second million of paperback sales, *The House of God* continues to afford medical students the shock of recognition, and to offer them comfort and amusement in the midst of their Hippocratic travails.

NOTES

An introduction to the 1995 edition, marking a million copies sold, of *The House of God,* by Samuel Shem, M.D.

Imagining the House of God

JACK COULEHAN

Not long ago I gave a workshop entitled "Imagining the House of God" at a conference for writers who were interested in exploring the medical experience. I began the workshop by asking each participant to describe the first image that came to his or her mind upon hearing the words "the house of god." Two of the twenty participants were physicians, one was a psychiatric nurse clinician, and the others were laypersons. One of the physicians, an oncologist from New Zealand, told us that she imagined a quiet spot in the giant fern forest near Franz Josef Glacier. Others reported images of sacred buildings, sites of natural beauty, or the interior life. Only two people immediately identified *The House of God* as Samuel Shem's satirical novel about medical internship. One was a family doctor from New Hampshire, and the other was the psychiatric nurse, who had not only read the book but also trained at McLain Hospital in Boston during the time Samuel Shem (Stephen Bergman) was a psychiatric resident there.

"He once asked me out," she told the group, but she wouldn't reveal her answer.

Since I've spent much of my career working with medical students and residents, I was surprised that only 10 percent of the audience was familiar with Shem's novel. This was a setback because I had intended to engage the group in taking an imaginative leap beyond the irony of the title and ask, "Is it possible that the dehumanized medical world of Shem's fiction might also have a spiritual dimension? Could the bitter satire of *The House of God* serve as a starting point for the moral imagination?" But to do that, they would have to know the story.

I had read *The House of God* as a young faculty member at the University of Pittsburgh medical school. The first sixty or seventy pages were hilarious, but after that I developed a creepy-crawly feeling that gradually grew and became overwhelming. I'm not sure if there is such a thing as false satire, or inauthentic parody, but that is how I thought of the book. While many of the characters and situations were recognizably "true" beneath the distortion and exaggeration, the overwhelming bitterness and pessimism seemed phony, or at least misdirected. I had the naive belief that the role of satire was to ridicule the status quo with the aim of improving it, but Shem's satire smashed everything in its path and left no survivors.

This reaction to *The House of God* was surprising because, like Roy Basch, I had quit my medical residency after the internship year due to dissatisfaction and alienation. Unfortunately, I had chosen one of the most academic residencies in the nation because the chief of medicine at my medical school had flattered me and urged me to do so. Lacking a clear sense of direction of my own, on June 25, 1969, I found myself in a ton of trouble at the Hospital of the University of Pennsylvania. When Dr. Arnold Relman, chair of medicine at Penn, rose to welcome the assembled interns, he told us we were the cream of the crop; a corps of elite Young Turks who would lead internal medicine into a new scientific era. My guts seized with terror because I was pretty sure that I wasn't a Young Turk. Relman had recently exiled most of the private attending physicians and reconstructed his department around a cadre of full-time researchers. After he spoke, the chief resident took over and told us about our every-third-night on-call schedule (every second night in the ICU) and our splendid opportunity to learn emergency medicine during six weeks of uninterrupted twelve-hour shifts at Philadelphia General Hospital. He concluded by reminding us that internship was both a joyous experience and a trial by fire. What had I gotten myself into?

After the initial terror, I settled into a tolerable routine. I enjoyed spending time with patients and their families but hated the atmosphere of competition and gamesmanship. Although unaware of it at the time, I also hated myself for not sharing the passion for medical science that animated my fellow interns. They lived and breathed adrenal hormones and distal tubules, while my interest in metabolism was purely adaptive. For the most part, attendings at Penn were supportive and devoted teachers. Naturally, I sucked up to them, buffed my image, covered my ass, and dropped references to current research whenever I could. But none of it felt right. I was putting in enormous effort to embark on someone else's journey. In my free time, I'd often sneak into the hospital library, where, for some reason, they had a large collection of travel books about exotic countries like India, Bhutan, Tahiti, Morocco, and Paraguay. In that way I began trying to find my own journey.

One day I screwed up my courage and told Dr. Relman that I was going to leave Penn at the end of the internship and take a job at an inner-city clinic in Pittsburgh. "Coulehan, you're making a big mistake," he told me. Then he explained that it would be unprofessional to quit, since I had supposedly committed to the full three-year program. Finally, he told me, quite calmly, that in the future, when I regretted the decision and returned with my tail between my legs, he wouldn't take me back. After a several-year detour in community medicine, I eventually completed my residency, but in another state at a more easy-going hospital. Thus, as a genuine post-internship dropout myself, why did I find Roy Basch's story so off-putting?

When I recently reread *The House of God,* the answer came crashing home. The book's dark humor is still effective, although now a bit tired, because Shem's funniest ideas have entered everyday medical discourse and are no longer surprising. Since its publication in 1978, *The House of God* has become a rite of passage for generations of premedical and medical students. While the grassroots consider it the definitive satire of internship, the ivory tower condemns it as heterodox. In my experience, *The House of God*'s irony and cynicism resonate with many students' expectations of clinical training. As these students approach the hospital, the book reinforces their image of the real world of medicine. Gallows humor, which at times may have a barely legitimate role in stress reduction, becomes glorified as a royal road to survival. In this way *The House of God* co-opts students into believing that internship is more about entitlement than patient care. In fact, the most distinctive and destructive feature of Shem's novel is that it parodies patients as much as or more than it parodies doctors.

Before I discuss the negative influence of *The House of God* further, a few caveats are in order. First, I'm not advocating censorship or book burning. Put *The House of God* on your reading list if you want to, no problem, but allow plenty of time for discussion and reflection. Second, I enjoy satire and, God knows, medical education provides plenty of targets for satire. Finally, I'm aware that my reading of *The House of God* is probably different from the author's intended meaning. I have no idea whether or not Shem intends for the reader to conclude, as I do, that Roy Basch is an immature narcissist whose lack of compassion antedates his internship, a conclusion that undermines much of what Roy tells us as a narrator.

The most striking dynamic in *The House of God* is the discrepancy between Roy's self-serving belief that he is a victim and the textual evidence that he is more perpetrator than victim. While he blames his dehumanization on the cumulative horrors of internship, the narrative shows little or no evidence of a slippery slope, at least as far as his attitude toward patients is concerned. He never even tries to care for them.

As he recuperates with Berry on a beach in France, Roy reflects, "Before the House of God, I had loved old people. Now they were no longer old people, they were gomers, and I did not, I could not love them anymore" (Shem 5). In fact, it's difficult for him to get emotionally close to anybody, even his naked and nubile lover. She reassures him that there are no gomers on the beach, so it's safe for him to stop being so guarded, but Roy cries out, "They can still hurt me" (8). More than three hundred pages later, Roy describes an epiphany that he has when Berry and the two emergency department cops have almost forcibly dragged him from the hospital to a performance by Marcel Marceau. As he enters the mime's imaginative world, Roy experiences a flash of insight:

"All of a sudden I felt as if a hearing aid for all my senses had been turned on. I was flooded with feeling. I roared. And along with this burst of feeling came a plunging, a desperate clawing plunge down an acrid chasm toward despair. What the hell had happened to me? Something in me had died. Sadness welled up in my gut and burned out through the slits of my eyes" (326). Shortly thereafter, he summarizes his experience: "This internship—this whole training—it destroys people" (328).

But this supposed self-discovery doesn't facilitate healing. Roy remains detached and traumatized. Will he be restored to a more humane state by Berry's all-forgiving love or by his career switch to psychiatry? Before we sympathize with his victimhood, let's look back to his first day of internship. Shortly after 6:30 A.M. Roy meets his soon-to-be mentor, the Fat Man, who tells him the team won't be making rounds to see the patients but rather will be flipping three-by-five index cards in the on-call room. "In internal medicine," the Fat Man says, "there is virtually no need to see patients. Almost all patients are better off unseen" (27). When Roy does encounter the gomers, he is disgusted by them. Before the end of his first day, he labels one patient a "heifer" and another a "hippo." The supposedly compassionate young doctor comments, "All of a sudden I thought 'zoo', that this was a zoo and that these patients were the animals" (32).

So Roy was already detached from patients on day one. The single glimpse of empathy we see is in his care of Dr. Sanders, a retired physician dying of lung cancer. Perhaps because of their similar backgrounds, Roy connects with Sanders as a suffering person and treats him humanely. The only other time that he directly responds to a patient's plight, his response results from anger, not compassion. After a fellow intern commits suicide, Roy "listens" to Saul, a patient with terminal leukemia who has requested euthanasia. Roy initially refuses but later storms into Saul's room and kills him with potassium chloride. In fact, throughout *The House of God* patients serve primarily as obstructions. Shem litters them across his hospital landscape like ridiculous, demanding, pathetic, and even malignant objects. They exist only to victimize Roy, Chuck, Potts, Eat My Dust Eddie, and the other house officers. Roy is so convinced of this victimhood that he doesn't even try to construct a narrative that convincingly shows its evolution.

Ironically, Roy's mentor, the Fat Man, reveals himself as the one compassionate physician in the hospital. Early in the book, Fats appears to be a savvy but unsympathetic resident who has mastered the system to meet his own needs. He teaches that "almost all patients are better off unseen" (27) and "these fingers do not touch bodies unless they have to" (28). We encounter him at the nursing station, sitting with his feet up and reading the *Wall Street Journal,* a prophet proclaiming the sardonic laws of the House of God. The man is hard headed, detached, subversive, and destined for a prestigious fellowship. Roy immediately adopts this version of Fats as his role model—or, more than that, his savior.

However, little by little, Fats reveals the person beneath his persona. First, Roy learns that the Fat Man's clinic overflows with patients who gravitate toward him because he listens to them: "These people didn't give a damn about their diseases or 'cures'; what they wanted was what anyone wanted: the hand in their hand, the sense that their doctor could care" (194). On another occasion, Roy is astounded to see Fats spending an hour comforting a woman to whom he has just given bad news. And after Potts's suicide, Roy reports, "The Fat Man was crying. Quiet tears filled his eyes, fat wet tears of desperation and loss. They rolled down his cheek" (284). The revelation that his role model has a human side agitates and alienates Roy, who lashes out in anger, exclaiming to Berry that "he's acting like a Boy Scout" and "he's not cynical enough. He's turned into a patsy. It's almost like he's deserting me" (252). Berry responds, "He hasn't killed off the caring part of himself. You have" (269).

However, Fats is no paragon of virtue. He exploits VA patients by enrolling them in research projects without their consent. He also teaches his disciples to falsify medical records ("buff" the charts) when it is in the patients' best interest not to have invasive procedures. In fact, the Fat Man is a complex character who doesn't fit the expectations created by this sledgehammer of a parody. The other characters are all two dimensional, with the possible exception of Potts, who needs slightly more texture to perform his role as sacrificial lamb. But the Fat Man is a genuine person.

Roy presents the data about Fats but finds it more confusing than enlightening. He never raises the question, Why hasn't the House of God destroyed the Fat Man, if it has destroyed so many others? Nor does he fully grasp the Fat Man's philosophy of "doing nothing," except perhaps as a survival technique that makes life less complicated and more efficient. However, for Fats, "doing nothing" represents working in the patient's best interest, while "medical care" is associated with only the doctor's self-interest. The Fat Man summarizes his beliefs in the thirteenth law, THE DELIVERY OF MEDICAL CARE IS TO DO AS MUCH NOTHING AS POSSIBLE. His disciples may view this as a statement about survival, but in fact it articulates a deep truth about illness and healing.

In the orthodoxy of *The House of God,* the alternative to doing nothing (i.e., "medical care") is the compulsion to cure by doing everything possible in any given situation. This results not only in more harm than good, but often in no benefit whatsoever, especially in chronically ill and elderly patients. Thus, "medical care" is the direct antithesis of the Hippocratic maxim, "At least, do no harm." Medical intervention doesn't prolong life since gomers never die, but it does cause complications that prolong hospitalization. Alternatively, younger, healthier people actually do sometimes develop fatal diseases or become victims of trauma. Unlike gomers, these patients can die, but Roy has little to say about treating them. Rather, he projects the fatalistic view that medical care makes little difference.

Jo, the resident who replaces the Fat Man as Roy's team leader, is a champion of invasiveness. Like Leggo, the chair of medicine, and Fish, his chief resident, Jo embodies a concept of medical care as aggression. Upon first taking charge of the unit, she tells Roy, "I never do nothing. I'm a doctor. I deliver medical care" (88). She insists on doing whatever *can* be done, regardless of whether it *should* be done. The Fat Man places Jo's beliefs in context: "The profession is a disease. It doesn't care what sex you are. It can trap us, any of us, and it's pretty clear that it's trapped Jo" (92). While it quickly becomes obvious to Roy and most of his fellow interns that the less aggressive you are, the better it is for the elderly patient, the hospital hierarchy can't accept this. As she rotates into the intensive care unit, Jo asserts, "I want to make one thing perfectly clear: we are going to win this war against death" (312).

The Fat Man uses the same metaphor but frames the antagonists differently. In his mind, the war takes place within the profession itself: it is not about doctors fighting disease in patients, but rather doctors fighting a disease in themselves— the compulsion to cure. "I'm telling you that the cure is the disease," he says. "The main source of illness in this world is the doctor's own illness: his compulsion to try to cure and his fraudulent belief that he can. It ain't easy to do nothing, now that society is telling everyone that the body is fundamentally flawed and about to self-destruct" (193).

As our narrator, Roy either cannot or will not tell us how medicine *should* be taught, in lieu of the teaching he parodies. However, from the data at hand, we infer that good medicine involves at least empathy, kindness, responsiveness, respect, advocacy, emotional openness, and even a smidgeon of physical contact, despite Fats's canard about not touching patients unless you have to. The Fat Man may preach detachment, but he demonstrates compassion. Fats is alienated from the medical hierarchy and what it represents, but he isn't alienated from patients, and that is precisely why his humanity has survived, while Roy's hasn't. (Notice that Roy sees himself as too dehumanized to demonstrate any of these qualities, which makes him angry with Fats.)

Alienation is the name of the game in *The House of God*. Interns lose their souls (i.e., become estranged from themselves and "destroyed") rather than becoming humane doctors. But why is the hospital experience so devastating? One possibility is that patients' demands, especially those of gomers, are just too overwhelming for anyone. Interns are Sisyphus-like creatures who endlessly carry their gomers up a slope, only to slide down and start again. In this scenario, interns are vulnerable, victimized, and inevitably drained. Another possibility is that this is the nature of aggressive medicine itself, whether practiced by the hospital hierarchy in the name of science or by private doctors in pursuit of money. Caught in the crossfire between these forces, house officers adopt a culture of survival: "Most of us had learned enough about medicine to worry less about saving patients and more about saving ourselves" (132).

A third possibility is poor physical working conditions. In the decades since *The House of God* appeared, residency reform has focused on decreasing residents' working hours, improving on-call schedules, and avoiding sleep deprivation among residents. There is evidence that such measures decrease dissatisfaction, depression, and medical error (Lockey, Cronin, et al.). However, *The House of God* doesn't parody working conditions as such. The Fat Man's laws make the interns' work more efficient but do so under the aegis of avoiding harm or futility, rather than setting up better standards for the work environment. In any case, the characters have plenty of time to enjoy casual sex in the on-call room and drink ginger ale at the nursing station.

Toward the end of the novel, Roy finally identifies the main cause of alienation: physical and emotional abandonment by the attending staff. He concludes that interns in *The House of God* are dehumanized because of their bad role models. Their supposed mentors not only don't care for their own hospitalized patients but don't care for the house officers either. The trainees find themselves bereft of inspiration and direction. As Roy observes, "Each of us was becoming more isolated. The more we needed support, the more shallow were our friendships; the more we needed sincerity, the more sarcastic we became" (261). In one of the climactic moments of the novel, Roy tells his chief, "What we're saying is that the real problem this year hasn't been the gomers, it's been that we didn't have anyone to look up to" (363). And then Chuck puts his finger on the core of the problem: "How can we care for our patients, if'n nobody cares for us?" (364).

In the dysfunctional house staff community, communication dries up. Ultimately, the interns don't listen to one another any more than they listen to their patients. Instead, they pursue intense but superficial sexual liaisons or take their anger out on patients. The only apparent avenue to salvation is the exit door. Wayne Potts commits suicide in desperation. Roy reports, "I could not 'be with' others, for I was somewhere else, in some cold place, insomniac in the midst of dreamers, far far from the land of love" (287).

The House of God reminds me of a sentiment about bad doctors expressed in one of Thomas Percival's letters. Percival was a physician who practiced at the Manchester Infirmary in England late in the eighteenth century. In response to bickering and patient stealing among Manchester physicians, the hospital trustees asked Percival to codify a set of ethical standards to serve as a corrective.

He responded by creating a broad virtue-based system of professional conduct, drawing extensively on David Hume's theory of moral sentiments and Dr. John Gregory's lectures on medical ethics at the University of Edinburgh. In the first chapter of his book, *Medical Ethics* (1803), Percival enjoined physicians to "unite tenderness with steadiness" in their care of patients. He went on to describe the consequences of striving for objectivity and detachment at the expense of "tenderness," saying that such physicians inevitably develop a "coldness of heart" that makes them insensitive to human suffering. "This coldness of heart, this moral insensibility," he wrote, "should be sedulously counteracted before it has gained an invincible ascendancy" (31).

In Roy's case "coldness of heart" was evident from the beginning, which at least partially undermines Samuel Shem's thesis that internship is dehumanizing. Given what I know about undergraduate medical education, I'm tempted to visualize Roy four years earlier, when he entered medical school. I've known many such students who begin their training with an avowedly firm commitment to compassion and social justice, but who later claim they were dehumanized by medical school. Many of our students at Stony Brook write reflective practice journals during their clerkships and electives. Granted, those who choose to journal are a self-selected minority and, therefore, unrepresentative of their colleagues. But sentiments such as the following are reasonably common. "I have come to the humbling realization," wrote one student near the end of her fourth year, "that, as a physician, I cannot give to my patients what I as a patient wanted. . . . We have never been encouraged to look at the assumptions and feelings that the physician brings to the process. . . . I don't want to be reminded of my own arrogance. What made me think I could do it better than anyone else? I can't." Another student, who had been a social activist in college, ended her journal with these sentiments: "When I arrived in medical school, I was eager to get involved. I was excited about addressing important issues. . . . However, medical school is an utter drain. For two years lecturers parade up and down describing their own particular niche as if it were the most important thing for a student to learn. And then during the clinical years, life is brutal, people are rude, the hours are long."

Medical school and residency are certainly challenges to the trainee's self-image and character, but it is more accurate to fault these institutions for failing to nourish positive character traits (i.e., virtues) than to implicate them for actively destroying virtue. "Destruction" implies that students already possess the psychological, interpersonal, social, and spiritual qualities needed for doctoring, but negative forces drive them away. However, "failure to nourish" acknowledges the fact that medical education is itself a process of character formation.

Perhaps Roy took a wrong turn in medical school. In any case, he enters internship without having developed the habits of the heart he needs to be a good doctor. He lacks both tenderness and steadiness. He hasn't internalized professional values or made himself a reflective observer of his own and others' behavior. Had he done so, patients would have been more than targets of ridicule. In Shem's parody of the mistaken priorities of medical care, patients should have been the primary victims. Even in a satire focused narrowly on internship as trial by fire, patients should at least appear as co-sufferers and secondary victims. But in *The House of God* patients are part of the prosecution rather than the defense.

Roy's lack of steadiness is apparent in his narcissistic inability to deal with complex characters and motivations. Had he developed more insight, Roy might have understood that the destructive features of hospital culture are not the result of a stereotypically malignant hierarchy ("the essence of any hierarchy is retaliation" [Shem 125]) as he imagines but rather of systemic failures that can, and often do, compromise well-intentioned physicians. When the Fat Man reveals himself to be a multifaceted human being, Roy rejects his mentor's tenderness, which at the same time makes him skeptical of the Fat Man's steadiness as well. In this parody of a hero's quest for salvation, Roy fails. All he can do at the end is lick his wounds and whine, since he rejects both objectivity ("medical care") and subjectivity ("doing nothing") in doctoring.

In the thirty years since *The House of God* appeared, medical educators have zeroed in on aspects of training that contribute to failures like Roy's. As physicians, we still visualize ourselves as members of a profession grounded in virtue and character, but modern medical institutions have generated a second clinical culture that incorporates values at odds with medical virtue. In the hospital setting, physicians may learn that behavior based on self-interest, detachment, and arrogance wins them more points than behavior based on altruism, compassion, fidelity, and humility, even though their physician role models may preach the latter. This illustrates a conflict between what medical educators *think* they are teaching (i.e., the explicit or formal curriculum) and what students and residents actually learn from immersion in hospital life (i.e., the tacit, informal, or hidden curriculum) (Coulehan). Everything we say that is designed to instill empathy, communication, compassion, trust, fidelity, and an investment in the patient's best interest constitutes the explicit curriculum. The hidden curriculum, consisting of our day-to-day practices, pushes these values aside and encourages objectivity, detachment, wariness, and distrust (Coulehan). Talking the talk is ineffective unless you also walk the walk. Take a look at Tom Inui's *A Flag in the Wind: Educating for Professionalism in Medicine* for a comprehensive analysis of this dynamic in clinical education.

To return to the workshop I mentioned at the beginning of this discussion, among the first questions the workshop participants asked were, "How has residency training changed since *The House of God* was written?" and "Is the story still relevant today?" One thing is for sure: the hospital in 2008 is an even more frenetic place than it was in 1978. The resident's patients are more frequently critically ill than was the case in the past, because stable patients are discharged much earlier now, and diagnostic workups and surgical procedures that once required hospitalization are performed in the outpatient setting. Residents have shorter working hours and less on-call time than in 1978, certainly a positive development, although it does lead to less continuity of care for their patients. There is also less continuity, and perhaps a lower level of general clinical skills among the attending staff because subspecialization, clinical research, and new pressures on reimbursement limit commitment to teaching. On the positive side, today's residencies take into consideration dimensions of doctoring other than medical knowledge and clinical procedures. The Accrediting Council for Graduate Medical Education requires that curricula address and evaluate so-called core competencies like interpersonal skills, professionalism, and the social context of medical care. Moreover, the resident's need for professional and personal support is widely recognized.

I suspect that these changes are beside the point when it comes to assessing the continued relevance of *The House of God*. In fact, Samuel Shem could well have written the same book about his experience had he completed his internship in 2007. Residency training has evolved, but its personal, professional, and spiritual challenges remain as great as ever, which is why *The House of God* continues to have a negative influence on medical education.

The problem is that the novel uses powerful existential themes in contemporary society (e.g., narcissism, isolation, entitlement, victimhood) to effectively debunk medical education. Students tend to internalize the message that clinical training is dehumanizing without sufficiently noticing that the group most dehumanized in the novel is patients. Its satire is easily assimilated into the "hidden" curriculum that exists in tension with humanizing elements of medical training. The most important of these, of course, is the opportunity to care for suffering patients as fellow individuals. *The House of God* tells students that it is impossible to do so. It also validates students' sense of victimhood by blaming institutions and hierarchies (as well as patients) for their own increasing alienation. It glorifies gallows humor but avoids self-deprecating humor.

Of course, the greatest irony of all is the book's title, a feature I had hoped to explore in the writing workshop. Just as Roy's journey through internship is a parody of the hero's quest for salvation, the House of God itself is a parody of a sacred space. Shem sets the stage on page 13 when he explains that the hospital was "founded in 1913 by the American people of Israel" so that their "medically qualified sons and daughters" could get good internships, otherwise unavailable to them "because of discrimination." Laudable though this may be, note that even here the goal is neither spiritual nor other directed. The House of God was created to benefit its doctors. If anything, its hierarchy suggests the structure of a church (thus more Christian than Jewish in this case) from which God is absent. The ultimate purpose of its prayers and ceremonies has been forgotten, but the hierarchy perpetuates them to meet its own needs—ambition, power, celebrity, and financial gain. The residents are acolytes who function as tools of these secular priests.

In parodying the spiritual dimension of medicine and the quest for meaning in medical practice, *The House of God* leaves Roy Basch and the book's readers in an isolated, helpless state. Where to next? How can I overcome these obstacles? Is it possible to become a good doctor in today's world? Too often medical educators shirk their responsibility to address these questions. Too often we ignore the dynamics of character formation in medicine and allow our students and house officers to develop coldness of heart in place of tenderness and steadiness. Too many students become resigned to Roy Basch's sense of loss, as evidenced in their journals by remarks like "As a physician I cannot give to my patients what I as a patient wanted" and "What made me think that I could do it better than anyone else?"

Our students and young physicians—not to mention our patients—deserve a better fate than *The House of God* deals them. Fortunately, many of them develop the qualities and skills they need to overcome that fate. Take, for example, this student who wrote near the end of her journal, "I never thought I would say such a thing—I'm going to miss medical school. It has been a wonderful experience for me, although painful at times. It is a privilege to pursue a career that you love—so many people can't say that they love their job. I am looking forward to the years ahead of me. I am truly happy." Roy Basch could learn a thing or two from her.

WORKS CITED

Accreditation Council for Graduate Medical Education. *ACGME Outcomes Project 7* July 2007 <http://www.acgme.org/Outcome>.

Coulehan, J. "Today's Professionalism: Engaging the Mind, but Not the Heart." *Academic Medicine* 80 (2005): 892–98.

Inui, Thomas S. *A Flag in the Wind: Educating for Professionalism in Medicine.* Washington, D.C.: Association of American Medical Colleges, 2003.

Lockey, S. W., J. W. Cronin, et al. "Effect of Reducing Interns' Weekly Work Hours on Sleep and Attentional Failures." *New England Journal of Medicine* 351 (2004): 1829–37.

Percival, Thomas. *Percival's Medical Ethics.* Ed. Chauncey D. Leake. New York: Robert E. Krieger, 1975.

Shem, Samuel. *The House of God.* New York: Dell, 2003.

Writing the Medical Training Experience in 1978 and 2006: *Body Language in* The House of God

STEPHANIE BROWN CLARK, NEETA JAIN, AND DAGAN COPPOCK

PART ONE BY STEPHANIE BROWN CLARK

Stephen Bergman was a writer before he was a doctor.

He began writing as a Rhodes scholar enrolled in a PhD program in physiology at Oxford in 1966. After two years of research on the neurophysiology of memory, Bergman realized that he did not want to be a scientist, but a writer. The U.S. involvement in the escalating war meant that Bergman would have to choose between Vietnam and Harvard Medical School. He imagined that medicine would be his meal ticket, and he would find a way to write. He graduated from medical school in 1973 and completed a one-year general internship at Beth Israel Hospital in Boston before his psychiatry residency. In 1974 he started writing *The House of God*. After seven rewrites, it was published in 1978.

As Bergman observes, he and his fellow interns were "products of the 60s, brought up on the civil rights movement and the Vietnam War" (934). In the novel, the survival of the interns, and their patients, depends on their recognition that the war on disease does not follow the prescribed rules of engagement, but the subversive laws of the House. The laws, devised by the Fat Man, a veteran in his second year of residency, deploy the tactics of guerilla warfare, based on intelligence, deception, and sabotage to undermine an authority through long low-intensity confrontation. The enemy is not the patient, but the inscrutable medical system in which both the patients and providers must operate. Bergman's novel reflects the era in which he came of age, in ways paralleling Joseph Heller's accounts in *Catch-22* a generation earlier. Bergman admits that the effect of these events on him and his writing was an insight that occurred to him in retrospect: "I had little or no idea of the unseen historical forces shaping me" (934).

While Bergman acknowledges several key historical forces that shaped him and his writing, there are other events in medical education in general, and in the academic discipline of literature and medicine in particular, that coincide with Bergman's personal development as physician and writer in the 1960s and 1970s. The institutional beginnings of the discipline of literature and medicine within emergent medical humanities programs in medical schools at this time would legitimize the value of medical narratives written by patients and by physicians about their experiences and create a place for the study of these literary works in academic medicine.

In 1967, at the time Bergman was beginning to write at Oxford, the first department in humanities at the new medical school at Penn State University at Hershey admitted its first students. At the time that Bergman was deciding on his own future, a group of clinicians, humanists, and social scientists formed the Society for Health and Human Values and convened their first meeting in Cincinnati.[1] With funding from the National Endowment for the Humanities, the Society for Health and Human Values, through its Institute on Human Values in Medicine, held a series of meetings that were attended by theologians, literary scholars, social scientists, writers, and physicians intent on integrating the humanities into medical training. The mission of the society reflected widespread reforms in medical education in the United States. In 1972 the new discipline of literature and medicine was introduced into a few medical schools. Literary scholars were being appointed to medical schools, and the study of literary texts and methods was introduced in their curricula (Charon 24). In its annual report on medical education for 1978–79, the AMA noted that 89 of 119 schools surveyed had formal programs in medical humanities, and 7 other schools were planning to do so (Bruer and Warren). The same year, the Modern Language Association convened its first special session on literature and medicine as a subdiscipline of literary studies.

The emergence of medical humanities programs that included courses on literature and medicine was in part a corrective in medical education to address the competing demands to teach an expanding body of scientific knowledge enmeshed in sophisticated technologies with the empathetic, attentive humanistic skills that comprise the "art" of medicine. Medical training needed to be directed not just at the understanding and treatment of the disease but also at the care of the patient.[2]

In 1978, at about the time *The House of God* was published, a group of academics published a slim volume on *The Role of the Humanities in Medical Education*. In it, Edmund Pellegrino observed that medical humanities have "achieved the status of a salvation theme which can absolve the perceived sins of modern medicine." The list of those sins is long and includes "over specialization, technicisms, over-professionalisation, insensitivity to personal and socio-culture values, too much curing and not enough caring, overmedicalization of everyday life . . . inhumane treatment of medical students, overwork by house staff." Medical humanities and its implicit humanism is "really a plea to look more closely at what medicine *should be,* and increasingly seems not to be." The "should be" is what ought to guide physicians and patients as they "are ushered through the techniques, mystiques, and bureaucracies that constitute modern medicine" in order to avoid the "humiliation and degradation of our humanity, so often built into the process" (Pellegrino 2).

Published in the same year, Bergman's book is the fictional enactment of the process, as Roy and his fellow interns and their patients are ushered through modern medicine's techniques, mystiques, and bureaucracies in the House of God. The appearance of *The House of God* was hardly auspicious. According to its author, "it had the worst publishing history of any book ever published." There were no advertisements, no reviews, no interviews. "The NYT was on strike so it didn't get reviewed there. It started selling by hardcover and then all the books were destroyed by a flood in a warehouse in NJ." It was discussed briefly and heatedly in the letters column of the *New England Journal of Medicine*. Some readers were shocked by the contemptuous treatment of chronically ill patients and senior physicians; others were impressed by the candor and accuracy of the author's portrayal of modern medicine.

The first review of *The House of God* appeared in 1982 in the first issue of *Literature and Medicine,* a scholarly journal devoted to the study of literary representation of illness, medicine, suffering, and healing. Titled *Towards a New Discipline*, the collection of essays presented a "tentative approach to the union of literature and medicine" and included a review of "Recent Works of Interest" by Peter W. Graham. Graham noted that the book "may offend fastidious readers" with dialogue that is "too faithful to be easily endured":

> Everything about the book—the alternating cheap cynicism and soggy romanticism, the sex, rage, horseplay, violence and squalor—may seem overdone. But the exaggerations of *The House of God,* like the medical caricatures of Hogarth and Rowlandson, convey rather than conceal truth. . . . For all its stridency the book speaks with conviction, and sometimes eloquence of a formative year that for real interns as well as Shem's fictional ones is likely to be too full of personal dilemmas and medical crises, a year when talented young people lose their illusions and learn bitter lessons—that medicine too rarely cures . . . that the path to becoming a "good doctor" can destroy a good person. (Graham 49)

Roy narrates the unhealthiness of his medical training experience in the House of God as if it were an illness experience or pathography. Although Roy's body is supremely healthy, he suffers a kind of soul sickness. He is wounded by the patients whom he cannot cure:

> Roy: I never did anything to hurt them, and they're trying to hurt me.
> Fat Man: Exactly, that's modern medicine. (Shem 96)

Roy ruminates on his "ridiculous diseased life" while he is caring for Dr. Sanders, a fifty-one-year-old physician on the staff "with a history of parotid and pituitary tumors and horrible complications" (92).

> I thought of Dr. Sanders, who would die, and of the gomers, who would not, and I tried to figure out what was illusion and what was not. I had expected just like in the *How I Saved the World without Dirtying My Whites* book, to have been rushing in and saving people at the last moments. . . . If there had been a feeling of power in the empty corridor at night and in the crowded elevator during the day, there had also been the awesome powerlessness in the face of the gomers and the helpless incurable young. . . . In months Dr. Sanders would be dead. If I knew I were to die in months, would I spend my time like this? Nope. My mortal healthy body, my ridiculous diseased life. (97–98)

Typically, "pathography" refers to patients' narratives about their personal and medical experiences of an illness. The narrative serves as a means to refashion a life wounded or disrupted by illness or disability and locates illness stories within a larger framework of medical discourse and cultural practice. Increasingly the wounded storyteller is not only the patient, but also the physician. For both patients and physicians, the telling of their stories is healing: "Stories repair the damage that illness has done to the ill person's sense of where she is in life and where she is going" (Frank 53). Stories heal physicians as well.

Despite the pervasive academic and professional disdain for *The House of God*, it remains an "underground classic" (Jones 734) that has achieved a "cult status" (Wear 496) for trainees. Despite awkward silence in literary criticism, the novel's infamous language ("gomer," "buff," "turf") and its laws of the House are embedded in medical culture. As one physician recalled, he had initially resisted reading it throughout medical school: "I thought I wasn't a cynical doctor. But when I read it at the end of fourth year, I thought, well basically, my life is this book" (Marston).

Thirty years on, *The House of God* still speaks to physicians-in-training. And the laws of the House that so many have found distasteful, unethical, and despicable paradoxically continue to resonate with many medical students and residents. Like Stephen Bergman, both Neeta Jain and Dagan Coppock were writers before they were doctors. They were interns during the writing and editing of the book *Body Language: Poems of the Medical Training Experience*, which was published in 2006, almost thirty years after *The House of God*. Their reasons for writing about medical training experience are in line with Stephen Bergman's—resistance, catharsis, a way to find meaning. For them, it is the laws of the House of God that reverberate the deepest.

PART TWO BY NEETA JAIN AND DAGAN COPPOCK

The experience of medical training can generate intense emotional responses in its participants. At its essence, *Body Language* is a collective journal, an anthology of poetic entries documenting these reactions, snippets of excitement, despair, insecurity, fear, sadness, horror, and humor. Bergman has commented that he initially wrote *The House of God* for "catharsis, to share with my buddies what had been the worst year of our lives" (936). Thirty years later, the same forces moved us to create *Body Language*. As an exercise in catharsis, it too made the burden of human suffering and the exhaustion of medical training more bearable.

Body Language arose from the remarkable observation that many medical trainees had sought poetry as an outlet of expression. The focused, intense language of poetry lent itself well to the focused, intense nature of medical training. Observing this, we wondered what would happen if we collected poetry from medical trainees at all levels and then arranged the poems chronologically. We predicted the narratives of each individual poet would come together as a powerful meta-narrative. Through many voices, a collective, universal voice might arise.

As we collected and edited the poems that would finally become *Body Language,* we found the emerging story to be enlightening and beautiful in ways we had not predicted. Certainly, we were surprised at the universality of the individual poems. However, the poems spoke with and informed each other. They were synergistic. Together, they nicely told the collective story of medical training—*our* story.

Thirty years after its publication, *The House of God* remains a remarkable novel. Its power exists because it perfectly and universally captures the experience of medical training. Though the specifics of medical care and hospital organization have changed, it knows the burden and beauty of caring for the infirm. It captures the intermittent triumphs and absurdities of humans fighting illness and death. The Fat Man has codified the absurdity for us.

The Fat Man's laws are the scaffold upon which *The House of God*'s narrative hangs. Many of the poems from *Body Language* echo and expound upon the laws of the House. Our own experiences as medical trainees since the publication of *Body Language* have evoked some personal reflections on the laws. For the sake of the essays below, we have divided the laws between us—Neeta Jain (NJ) and Dagan Coppock (DC). We have subsequently interwoven excerpts from *The House of God* with our own experiences as residents. In this way, thirty years after Roy Basch, we will contemplate the connection of our own trials with trials that occurred before we were born.

THE FAT MAN'S LAWS REVISITED

I. Gomers don't die. (NJ)

Rotikansky was an old basset. He'd been a college professor and had suffered a severe stroke. He lay on his bed, strapped down, IVs going in, catheter coming out. Motionless, paralyzed, eyes closed, breathing comfortably, perhaps dreaming of a bone, or a boy, or a boy throwing a bone. . . . Turning to Fats, I said, "This is too sad. He's going to die."

"No, he's not," said Fats. "He wants to, but he won't."

"He can't go on like this."

"Sure he can. Listen, Basch, there are a number of LAWS OF THE HOUSE OF GOD. LAW NUMBER ONE: GOMERS DON'T DIE." (Shem 34)

The Fat Man's edicts are laws of nature. They are immortal. After a rotation in San Francisco's county emergency department as an intern, I wrote down a memory of one of my patients. I think it illustrates this particular law's resilience:

I remember a man, an old, crumpled man on a gurney in the emergency department pressed up against the wall like a tattered leaf wet against a curb in late autumn, skin veined with tattoos and wrinkles. He called the ambulance himself, short of breath with end-stage lung cancer. The first thing he tells me is "I love my wife. I want to go home." His chest X-ray confirms a sheet of white fog where a left lung should float. His skin shines green, canvassed with tattoos delicate in their depictions of slaughter: thick-muscled men with lines for biceps and triceps next to women with Barbie doll bra sizes and long hair.

This hardened man with stencils of knives and blood on his back refuses a lung tap to help him breathe more easily and pulls his urine-stained sheet closer. "I want to be with my wife." With conviction, he pulls himself up to go. I last see him holding himself through his zipper, dribbling small splashes of urine down the hall, about to walk into another patient's room looking for the exit.

II. Gomers go to ground. (DC)

We told them as ghost stories—the legends of residents who couldn't hack it, who dropped out, who made terrible mistakes. And like all good ghost stories, the stories of lost residents were vague, though imbued with enough details to make them real, or plausible. Their mistakes could have been mine; they could have been anyone's.

In *The House of God,* the hospital humiliated its residents for their mistakes. However, since the book was published, medical training has largely lost its element of humiliation. True, there are still older physicians who carry on the tradition of cruelty, but those old-guard attendings are becoming extinct. External humiliation is now being replaced by internal shame. In a career driven by overachievers, present-day residents are the architects of their own self-loathing. For every Yellow Man for whom residents have made a poor decision, there is still a Leggo or chief resident there, if only in the residents' own minds, ready to shame.

Recently, I discussed this concept with one of my program's benevolent administrators. "Shame," he told me, "is not always a bad thing. In fact, that's how we choose you. We pick residents who are going to be hard on themselves. Shame can build as well as it can destroy. In the end we have to do little policing, beyond occasional constructive feedback. Residents police themselves—when they look into the mirror or into each other's eyes."

To serve that function of policing, there are the aforementioned "ghost stories." They are cautionary tales in the truest sense. Their lesson was always the same. Implicitly, they say, "If you are having trouble, personal or otherwise, that's okay, but you must seek help." The question remains: is help waiting? When doctors are ill, who will care for them?

Body Language is filled with stories of emotionally strained physicians. In these stories, personal lives intersect subtly, sometimes dangerously, with professional lives. Mairi Leining's "October 1st" is exemplary of one such intersection:

You ask about my day—
I should have taken a Polaroid:
lime curtains, black sheets
yellow man, your age
rusted nails on restless fingers
pregnant belly with twisted purple veins
afraid to ask for directions.

Said he drank to escape the loneliness
That down escalator, no basement floor

I hold his hand, breathe through my mouth
discuss the facts from yesterday's spill;
a new liver, perhaps

You ask about my day—
I tell you it was fine;
my side of the bed grows further.   (Jain, Coppock, and Clark 112)

In this poem a marriage is failing from the distance created by the hospital. Will the failing marriage impair the physician? At what point will personal discord affect a doctor's ability to treat and give attention to his or her patients? My intern year, a story was told around the residents' lounge. It was about a senior resident, two months shy of graduating, who was kicked out of the program. I cobbled together his complete story from many late-night on-call retellings by older residents. It is difficult to know which details were true and which were apocryphal. He had been having "personal problems." These problems revolved around a relationship he had been struggling to maintain since his intern year. On an elective month, as a grand gesture, he left the country to tour France with his lover. This was, of course, a vacation not sanctioned by the program. By some accounts the risky nature of the move was meant to demonstrate, after years of residency-related neglect, a renewed commitment to his lover. For the sake of his relationship—and to prove a point—he planned to shirk all responsibility for a month.

As he was on an elective, that responsibility was minimal. His presence was not essential, and his absence was initially unnoticed. However, he made one critical error. He forgot that, though he might not be missed in the hospital, he had a once-weekly clinic obligation. When he didn't show up for his clinic, the program paged him. For reasons that were unclear to those telling his story, he had brought his pager to France. When he returned the page from a strange foreign number, he was immediately busted. The program laid out a quick suspension, and he flew back from France in a panic. Ultimately, he was dismissed with little mercy. Or so the story went.

For several months after his dismissal, the older residents reported sightings of him. He was described as appearing ill. They said he looked thin, his skin pale. It was as if no longer being a doctor had made him less substantial, a ghost of his former self. On one occasion I even heard a senior resident refer to him as a gomer, directly referring to *The House of God*. I had never heard a resident say that of another resident. "And what do gomers do?" the senior asked me. Before I could respond, he answered his own question, "gomers go to ground."

III. At a cardiac arrest, the first procedure is to take your own pulse. (DC)
A few definitions are in order.

Cardiac arrest: the complete cessation of all activity of the heart.

Code blue: an intercom signal used in hospitals. It generally indicates cardiac arrest, though it is also used for other crisis situations, such as respiratory arrest and patient nonresponsiveness. Such a signal calls critical emergency personnel to a patient's bedside. When "Code blue!" is called over a hospital intercom, someone somewhere is dying.

Coding a patient: what an emergency team does when they gather for a code blue. When someone is trying to die, "coding" is the process of actively resisting death.

ACLS: advanced cardiac life support—the advanced system physicians, nurses, and EMTs use to save lives. To define ACLS, the American Heart Association has created a number of algorithms. They are prearranged pathways of thought designed to save lives and prevent panic in those saving lives.

One of the most striking features of *The House of God* is its blatant, unapologetic sexuality, usually between doctors and nurses, and often occurring in such life threatening situations as above. A common critique of the book is that its depiction of sex revels in certain hierarchies and is, as a consequence, sexist. The counterargument is that the depictions are, instead, a mere recording of a sexist period in American medicine and not sexist in and of themselves. Regardless of their view on this matter, what many readers find disturbing is the juxtaposition of sex with crisis.

In *Body Language,* Richard Berlin's poem "On Call, 3 A.M." negotiates the tension between sexuality and death:

After she pages me to pronounce him,
we pull the white sheet to his chin
in one quick movement, our eyes
on his, then locked on each other's.
We know what we want.
In the deserted call room
with its fresh linen and barren walls,
we smell each other in the darkness,
the sweat on our scrubs, antiseptic soap
on our fingers. We lick each other's salt
like deer ready to run the instant we are called.
We know how to strip a body fast,
our uniforms falling to the linoleum floor,
our pleasure like worn stones tumbling in the tide.
We know what pours from the sea
of our bodies will not be tested in the lab,
and what we say will not be recorded in a chart,
though our movements are as efficient
as any surgical procedure. And afterwards,
when we kiss and wash our hands again,
we smooth the sheets and pull them tight.
We even make hospital corners.   (Jain, Coppock, and Clark 101)

Though there is little information about the circumstances of this death, there is the sense of its inevitability. In that way, death is no different from sex or birth. In Berlin's poem, understanding such relationships is a critical piece of a resident's training. What we do not know is whether the death was gentle and expected or a harried code blue, one in which the characters frantically fought death.

It is my first code blue: all terror and subliminal cuts. Panic and run-on sentences.

The patient's heart rate, his blood pressure, cannot be measured.

Age fifty-eight.

My father's age.

The monitor shows ventricular fibrillation, one step to flatline.

"He has a pulse," the nurse shouts.

He is someone's father, I think and count the people in the room. Sixteen. They look at me for direction then look away when I say nothing.

The respiratory therapist points at me, says, "What do we do next?"

I remember my algorithm, open my mouth to speak, but someone shouts,

"His pulse is gone." On the monitor the patient's heart rhythm has organized to V tach then flipped back to nothing.

My algorithm is useless.

"He's not breathing!" shouts the intern.

"What do we do next?" I don't know who has shouted this. I am thinking of my own father, who is ill, five hundred miles away.

"Shock him," I say weakly.

"He's lost his pulse. We can't shock that!"

Ashamed, I again open my mouth to speak, and again nothing comes out.

An older nurse is drawing blood, says, "What do we do?"

"Who's in charge here? Is it you?" the anesthesiologist calls from across the bed.

"He's got a pulse," shouts a woman, a nursing student.

I am lost here. All knowledge slips away. I can only think of my father.

Only then do I feel her take my arm at the elbow.

"Someone needs to take charge here," the anesthesiologist shouts.

She is the other unit resident. She whispers, "Intubate him. Let him breathe, let's." She allows the sibilance, its warmth, to flow into my ear. I close my eyes. For a moment, I am gone. But I recover.

"Tube him," I shout. Anesthesia places the endotracheal tube.

Her hand slides down my forearm. She takes his wrist. I feel my own pulse beneath the pressure of her finger. "You're sweating," she says, then, "But now you're both breathing. Let's make his heart beat again. Epinephrine."

"Epinephrine one milligram," I shout.

He feels her breast brush against him as she draws even closer.

"You're doing just fine," she tells me.

"He's got a pulse, the rhythm's disorganized," someone says.

"Shock him," she says.

"200 joules. Everyone clear!" I am amazed at the authority in my voice.

The other resident and I back up. In the cramped room, our shoulders press back against the wall. Her palm takes mine, our fingers interlacing. "Clear!" the nurse shouts. The patient's chest jumps from the bed. His rhythm fades to nothing, then arises—a burst of electricity—alive, beating.

"Jesus," I say, my voice quiet. "I almost lost him." I can smell her shampoo. I think of sex, suppress it.

"You shouldn't feel ashamed," she says. "You saved his life."

IV. The patient is the one with the disease. (NJ)

The Fat Man warns his protégés of Law IV when they blame themselves for their patients' deterioration. Hapless Potts, second-guessing his patient management of a young father dead of a ruptured aneurysm, loses his self-esteem, confidence, and hope, ultimately committing suicide. "It was too late. If I had moved faster, maybe—The fatherly fat man pores into him: THE PATIENT IS THE ONE WITH THE DISEASE" (60).

The tendency to self-blame for poor outcomes makes us slaves to circumstances beyond our control. The Fat Man reminds us not to live the illnesses of our patients nor to blame ourselves for the multiple strikes of chance and fate that ultimately lead to a patient's demise.

And yet, one day at the end of my second year of residency, I found myself bearing this very burden and wrote:

Chief Complaint. His wife had long blond hair, curly, that tapered to the curve of her back. She looked younger than him. He was 73 with a full dark brown mustache. No gray. Maybe it was the mustache that did it. History of Present Illness. She didn't leave his side. Past Medical History. "The doctors say you need radiation to your brain, so that's just what we've got to do, right?" she'd say to him. Medications/Allergies. Shaving his face, she applied his cologne the day after his first treatment. She said it was Tuscany. Family History. I didn't understand her cheerleader spirit as if he was at the optometrist (his own profession) and not five days into a new diagnosis of metastatic lung cancer. Social History. Sometimes it's hard not to eavesdrop. Vital Signs. I heard her on the phone outside his room, hidden from view along the nursing station, her voice lifting. Physical Exam. "It's just devastating." Laboratory Values. "You've been a friend for so long." Assessment and Plan. "I don't know what we're going to do."

The gift of our medical training brings with it the helplessness of terminal illness. And it is the Fat Man who reminds us not to make it our own sickness, to avoid self-blame for tragedy beyond our control, not to carry the heavy stones of suffering in the pockets of our white coats.

V. Placement comes first. (NJ)

This law underscores the cynicism embedded in medicine, reflecting the frustration of caring for the old and infirm.

> "We are men of the law," said Quick, and we followed the House LAW: PLACE-
> MENT COMES FIRST, and called the Hebrew House. Alas, during the ambulance
> ride here, Anna O's bed was sold. (73)

Jerald Winakur's poem "He Still Whistles" offers a different perspective. It is the physician's reflex to offer placement as a management option to the wife of his demented patient. She refuses, encouraging us to loosen our cynicism and remember the life they lived together. It is their history that gives her the strength to care for him now.

They come every four months
he smiles, drools, sits quietly
always says yes, only says yes

she bitches and sighs, bemoans
and cries, He's getting worse
he's only getting worse. . . .

She can't take it anymore
and neither can I.
Have you considered a Home? I ask

prying into her blubbery folds
trying to discern what's inside
looking into her ruined

mascara-caked eyes
red and wrinkled now beyond relief
When she shyly says, Doctor,

I've gotten so fat . . . but do you know

he still whistles when
I take off my clothes . . .

and he sits there smiling, smiling
Grinning, nodding
Yes, he says. Yes.   (Jain, Coppock, and Clark 130)

VI. There is no body cavity that cannot be reached with a #14 needle and a good strong arm. (DC)

When patients think of the pain inflicted on them by physicians, needles are often what come to mind. Their thoughts go back to childhood inoculations—those times when they first offered up their skin to be broken—when one learned that pain can be for the greater good.

To physicians, a needle is one of the nicer discomforts we impose. Even at their largest gauge, needles are mere slivers of trauma. In the right hands, they can do their work, leaving minimal pain as they go. Doctors know they can do much worse.

In seeking out body cavities, there is perhaps no more noxious stimulus we deliver than the placement of a naso-gastric tube. Also known as NG tubes, they are our best access to the stomach. They allow for suction to pump out poisons. They remove the stomach's own acidic fluid, preventing aspiration. They relieve the pressure of an obstruction. They allow for tube feeding and pill administration when someone can't swallow on his or her own. Despite these advantages, they are exhausting for patients. To place them, the doctor must force the plastic NG tube, the width of a pinky, into the nostril. The tube must then, through shear force, be thrust over the nasopharynx into the oropharynx and down the esophagus. Along the way, this process triggers the body's need to sneeze and gag, which continues even after placement.

The trauma of placing these tubes is frequently felt, albeit to a much lesser degree, by the caregivers placing them. In the poem "NG Tube," poet Sarah Jane Cook describes the harrowing first experience of placing one:

Eyes watery and small.
A mouth full
of chalky growths and white ulcers,
mucous pooled.

We slip the greased tube into her right nostril,
blood begins to ooze.
I hear the first real words gurgle from

That mouth—
"Oh my god."

We can't get in.
We pull it out.
Tears drip down her
thin, drooping skin.

We try the other side.
Cough, gag,
it curls in the white pasty mouth.
Gag again, pull back.
Push,
it goes down.

She looks me in the eyes.   (Jain, Coppock, and Clark 81)

Just like Law VI, this poem reminds us that the fact that we *can* access doesn't necessarily mean we should. When does the harm we inflict on our patients outweigh the benefits? As an intern and resident, I often asked myself this question. One particular case comes to mind:

Thirty-five years old, Down syndrome, otherwise healthy. He looks me in the eyes. His are blue, trusting. I wonder what he sees in mine. I have often been told—by patients, by friends, by lovers—that my eyes give away everything.

I say, "You are bleeding from your bowels. We need to see what's inside. But first we need to clean your bowels. And it takes medicine to clean your bowels."

Can a doctor's eyes—can *my* eyes—simultaneously be kind and merciless?

"Since you couldn't drink the medicine on your own, we'll have to place this tube . . . to make you take your medicine."

The nurse whispers in my ear, "This will get ugly. It's going to take four-point restraints, I'm afraid. Of course, you'll have to put in the order."

"Will a verbal order count?"

"Of course."

"Then let's do it."

I raise the head of the patient's bed. I keep my eyes locked with his. The nurse hands me the NG tube. "Lean toward me," I say, pulling him forward, chin to chest. "Doctor," he says, "hi." I say "hi" back, move forward with the tube, the patient smiling, still my friend.

VII. Age + BUN = Lasix dose (DC)

Strange, specific, technical, mathematic . . .

The seventh law appears to be out of character with the other laws. In the novel, its utility certainly plays out. But it seems lazy, a law without art or wisdom. Because of its esoteric nature, it does not have, at first glance, the same potential universality of the other laws.

However, on a closer read, it contains two powerful lessons. The first: medicine, by its nature, tends to objectify patients. Our medical therapies and diagnostic tools are a marriage of science and technology applied to the vagaries of human existence and health. This is not to say that medicine should be abandoned. It's an excellent means of caring for the human body; but it cannot be forgotten that it has the potential to dehumanize.

The second lesson of the seventh law: medicine, at a certain point, becomes futile. For most of the patients in *The House of God*, quality of life has expired long before the patient does. Day-to-day care in the novel largely revolves around the proverbial rearranging of deck chairs on the *Titanic*. Fluid shifts and diuresis are often a major component of the human body's rearrangement. Law VII brings the nature of these acts into question. Its target is Lasix, one of our strongest diuretics, a remarkably resilient medicine since the days of *The House of God*.

Today, like thirty years ago, a huge component of fluid management is the foley catheter. The catheter is a plastic tube that, once inserted into the urethra, can ultimately access the bladder. It allows for accurate measurements of urine output, which can, in turn, be weighed against fluid intake. The poem "Foley" by Mindy Shah recounts a student's first foley placement:

As a kid you pissed
your name in the snow; at sixteen
you showed it to a girl
for the first time, face damp
and flushed. Now wires
thread your body.
I pull your old penis
from the fat seat of your thigh
and hold tight
as the catheter slides in to let
the blood and urine out,
tubing taped to your leg,
your glorious moment passed—
my first one.   (Jain, Coppock, and Clark 60)

The frankness of the poem borders on anger. It has a cynicism that rivals that of the seventh law. This will not be the speaker's last foley placement. It will not be the last foley the patient receives. Will the patient be saved because of it? Will his quality of life ultimately change for the better? It's hard to know, given the details of the poem. However, this poem and the seventh law are asking us to consider these questions. To what end do we treat? When do we stop?

VIII. They can always hurt you more. (NJ)

I believe it is a bombardment of disease coupled with a lack of time to process and recover from those hits that create the hurt and pain that afflict house staff. After a several-month stretch of difficult rotations, burnout evident, I wrote of my own fatigue in a journal:

> I do not smile for days. I feel a sullenness settle around me like a fog, stuck, stagnant, where the breeze does not blow, and I wonder of this training process that makes me mean, callous, that pushes me so much I feel numb, frozen. I feel like an automaton—a shell performing a job because the inside of me is not standing. It is hunkered within the body of me saying mercy—the game is over. I am done. I don't have the fight. And who is this person without patience, who does not have time for courtesy, who is full of anger and bitterness and frustration? Somewhere along the way I lost my kindness. It fell out of my pocket on my way to work. I knew it had been slipping toward the edge, just barely hanging out, but then when I felt the ice around my heart form, I knew it had fallen out, made a rainbow in a puddle and faded away. Something happened to make me mean and cold, and I think it was that the circumstances of my training were mean and cold to me.

This law of the Fat Man addresses house staff burnout. The experience I have described here is not unique to me. In multiple discussions with my peers, I have realized we have all faced varying degrees of the same sentiments, and thankfully, after rest and self-care, we recover. Sharing our experiences helps us get through. This exercise of shared experience is exactly what *Body Language* and *The House of God* accomplish, helping others through the arduous process of medical training. The following selections, the first from *The House of God,* and the second from *Body Language,* illustrate two reactions to being overwhelmed and exhausted. Roy's pain manifests as embarrassment and fatigue, while the senior in Richard Berlin's poem feels anger and a shell of numbness that breaks down into despair.

After his first night on call, one of Roy's patients has a heart attack. Roy does not have the emotional reserve to care for his patient or talk to her family. He reports:

I tried to persuade the intensive-care resident to take her off my service, but taking one look and saying, "Are you for real?" he refused the TURF. Sheepishly, trying to avoid the family, I slunk down the hallway. The Fat Man pointed out a valuable HOUSE LAW, NUMBER EIGHT: THEY CAN ALWAYS HURT YOU MORE. I finished my work for the day, and woozy, paged Potts, to sign out to him for the night. (Shem 82)

Richard Berlin's poem in *Body Language* called "January Thaw" serves as a correlate to Roy's experience in the House of God:

It is the winter of chest pain and snow,
all the drunks smashed
through the ER doors.

The Senior Resident in his new blue coat
can coax a silent heart,
but only curses the jaundiced men,

exiles them to frozen doorways,
shivered Thunderbird,
the lukewarm comfort of bitter coffee.

And he hates Drunken Johnny most of all,
loathes him and saves him,
Johnny rising immortal in disregard

for the slum of his body.
One night, he stumbles in, explosive,
ice loaded on his beard,

snow like soot falling from his flak jacket.
He shuffles to the gurney,
The Senior's rage like an ice storm.

Johnny's hands shake
to untie a glazed lace,
and when he grunts a drunken heave

on his boot, his foot breaks off

silent as torn moldy bread.
Johnny collapses, an intern vomits,

But the Senior stands hard
until tears kick across his face
and he wails like spring rain for a surgeon.   (Jain, Coppock, and Clark 105–6)

IX. *The only good admission is a dead admission. (DC)*

Intensive Care
by Mindy Shah

A get well soon balloon
hovers above the hiss
of the vent, calculated volumes
of gas to feed both
the balloon, your body.

Granddaughter's gift,
photos of the family
frame the rack
where the chart expands
with the epic of your death.

Pages dangle
where the holes
ripped through,
nobody bothers
to bind anything anymore.   (Jain, Coppock, and Clark 93)

Though not explicitly mentioned in the poem, the imagery and tone invoke
the mood of a CMO room. When patients are made CMO, by family members
or by health care proxies, their care has been shifted toward "comfort measures
only." Heroic attempts at sustaining life are ceased. All nonpalliative treatments
are withdrawn. Pain and anxiety relief become the focus. The plan is for a peaceful death. As is the case in "Intensive Care," a stillness seems to come over such
a room. The detritus of cards and gifts and flowers pays a strange homage to
the body at their center.

Patients tend to be made CMO in the ICU, the last and highest level of care
for the dying. But these patients cannot stay in the ICU forever. There is no

disrespect meant by this. More acutely ill people are arriving all the time, and ICU beds must be available. It is better for the patient to be moved to a quieter, less critical ward of the hospital. Patients are transferred to the floor so that families may grieve in a more peaceful environment and so that other patients may be treated in the ICU.

A CMO patient often moves at night, when the shuffling of patients between the ER, the wards, and the ICU is a delicate balance: every patient must be kept safe, but night staffing is limited. When they leave the ICU, CMO patients will often fill a ward bed that might otherwise have been filled by an emergency room patient. If the hospital is full, an ER patient must wait in the ER.

Overnight, when CMO patients arrive on the floor, the residents are happy. There is little work to be done with the patient. There is no intervention to be made. There will be no more code blues. No more shocks or CPR. And a hospital bed has now been filled. The residents' load has been lightened. With this smaller amount of work, maybe the resident will get some sleep.

Sometimes, in such situations, we feel guilty about the joy that arrives alongside a CMO patient. Maybe it is us at our worst. In truth, it is us at our weakest. It is us at our most tired, our most overworked. It is us thinking about our families, our children, our wives, our husbands—all home, asleep without us. The last gift of a dying patient becomes a gift to us—a moment of rest, a moment of reprieve.

XI. Show me a medical student who only triples my work and I will kiss his feet. (DC)

XII. If the radiology resident and the medical student both see a lesion on the chest X-ray, there can be no lesion there. (DC)

No one had felt the CT scan was necessary except the med student. She was convinced the scan would pick up a subtle cancer, one that was undetectable on our physical exam and previously obtained ultrasound. The attending, the interns, and I, as the resident, thought the patient had a simple case of gastroenteritis—an illness best treated with IV fluid and bowel rest. No need for wasteful high-tech studies.

Still, the medical student was persistent, and ultimately we did give in. The student was vehement, and the patient was not getting better. When the scan's read came in, I was shocked to find that the student was right. The patient's abdomen was filled with pathologic lymph nodes—metastatic cancer from some unclear source.

Before we could discuss the results, the student, triumphant in her diagnostic skills and confident in her empathy, entered the patient's room. She told the patient the diagnosis. She left the room crying.

I found her later, face red, bawling in the call room, and completely misread the situation.

"The patient must've been pretty broken up," I said. "I'm sure you broke it as gently as anyone could." I had completely misread the situation. I assumed that she and the patient had shared tears over the diagnosis, the medical student holding the patient's hand throughout.

Through the sobs, she confessed, "The patient yelled at me. She told me I was wrong and stupid. She said I was going to be a bad doctor."

As a student, you're stuck in an impossible situation. Your strongest desire is to please. Still, you are the target of every person in the hospital—the interns, the residents, the attendings, the nurses, the techs, the janitors. To become the target of the patient, the one about whom you most care, can be crushing.

After two years of residency, I was used to being shouted at. Patients handle shock and grief in all kinds of ways. Anger is just one of them. As a student, this hasn't had a chance to sink in. It takes time and experience to know that, once traumatic news is broken, a patient may respond with rage, may appear to hate you. Trainees often do not realize that the next day, once the anger has subsided, you may be loved again.

Pandora
by Kelley Jean White

September.
Second year medical student.
An early patient interview at the Massachusetts
General Hospital.
Routine hernia repair planned, not done.
Abdomen opened
and closed.
Filled with disease,
cancer.

The patient is fifty-six,
a working-man, Irish.
sit with him, notice the St. Christopher medal
around his neck.
"Can't hurt, can it?" he laughs.
I have become his friend.

I bring him a coloring book picture
that shows this thing, this unfamiliar organ
that melted beneath our hands
at dissection:
Pancreas.

Leaving his room, crying,
avoiding classmates,
I take the back stairs.
I find myself locked,
coatless, in the courtyard outside.
November.   (Jain, Coppock, and Clark 50)

So it goes when you are a student. Even when you connect, you feel locked
out, isolated. In that in-between period when you are "not quite a doctor," your
place in medicine and in life seems unclear.

As residents, we see our students going through these emotions. Often, because of our own busy schedules, we don't help our students as we should. But
there is another reason we don't help—a more selfish, callous reason. We know
that our students' sense of exclusion won't last forever. They will be inducted into
internship soon enough. And, regarding the trials of medical training, there is
much worse ahead.

X. If you don't take a temperature, you can't find a fever. (NJ)

XIII. The delivery of medical care is to do as much nothing as possible. (NJ)

These laws of the Fat Man are interrelated. In the House, Dr. Leggo, the chairman of
medicine, begins to grasp the Fat Man's laws, regarding the delivery of no medical
care as the most helpful action his interns could take for their patients.

"IF YOU DON'T TAKE A TEMPERATURE YOU CAN'T FIND A FEVER—
that's really trying your hardest to do something by doing nothing, right?"
"Right, Primum non nocere with modifications," I said. (162)

These laws remind me of one of my own patient encounters while I was an
intern on night float.

It started with a blasting page in the middle of the night. A nurse called to
report, "Mrs. C is short of breath, with O2 sats in the 80s." One line on a sign-out:
"82 year old female with a h/o A-fib with metastatic lung cancer. DNR, culture

if febrile." Contacts like cardboard, I blink and blink again. Can't find my sock. What if I didn't go? Would it just go away? Three terrified seconds later, I blink. Remind self to draw air into lungs. Pull on found sock. Here we go.

"Hi Mrs. C. How are you feeling?" Blink. Glasses unspotted, large, covering chin to brow. Hair dyed dark brown. No roots. I think about the three new gray hairs that just sprouted on top of my head. Focus, right.

She looks exhausted. "Mrs. C, how are you?" I ask again. She looks at me like I'm an idiot. Her silence says, "Isn't it obvious?" I feel like an idiot. When her nurse slips on the non-rebreather mask, she gives me a raised, disapproving eyebrow. Can she tell I'm new at this?

I get an EKG. A-fib, rate okay. I review the chest X-ray from a few hours earlier—maybe some CHF? She gets lasix. Now what?

I go back in, and she draws an outstretched index finger along her throat.

"Let me die."

She makes scissor signs with her fingers in the air as if she were cutting the cord.

Two milligrams morphine. Blink. No urine. It's been an hour now. Maybe it's not CHF and her sats are still low. Crap. PE?

"Mrs. C, I think to help you, we need to look at the blood vessels in your chest." She starts pushing the plunger of an imaginary air syringe she makes out of her fingers into her IV. No. "Let me die." She looks at me hard, and I know I am not the one giving orders tonight.

"Okay," I say. "I get it."

I call the attending. It's 3 A.M.

After a quick review of events, I ask, "Can we make Mrs. C comfort care? She's refusing the CT angio."

"Give her a dose of lovenox and we'll talk about it in the morning."

"But. . . ." Click.

Hi, Mrs. C. I'm back. We're going to give you this shot because . . . oh, whatever. I ask her nurse for two more milligrams of morphine. She breathes a little easier. She gets the lovenox too. I don't try to explain. But she gives me another scissor sign.

I check on her a little later. She eyes me. This time both eyebrows in line, she says, "You have courage."

I think I hear "courage" but am not sure. "I have what?"

"Courage."

"What's that again?"

"Courage."

I'm flustered. I do not understand and need her to repeat it three times.

"Courage for what, I ask?"

"You have courage, watching me die."

I don't know what to say, eventually stammering, "No, I'm watching you live."

I call her family and they come. Her multiple Italian progeny are tearful, demanding explanation. "She wants to die," I say. They too see she is ready and stop arguing. I slip away, taking her gift of courage.

She dies at ten o'clock the next morning.

CODA BY STEPHANIE BROWN CLARK

While the Fat Man's laws in *The House of God* reverberate with the experiences of physicians-in-training in *Body Language,* there are significant differences that reflect the historical forces that have shaped a new generation of physician-writers, like Neeta Jain and Dagan Coppock and their fellow poets thirty years on. Since 1978 much about the health care system and residency training has changed, including the length of hospital stays, the effects of managed care, and the implementation of a mandatory eighty-hour workweek for residents. In place of Vietnam and civil rights, the newer generation of physicians-in-training are products of the information age. Personal computers and the Internet have allowed connections and virtual communities to flourish. Joanne Trautmann's hardcover annotated bibliography of literature and medicine published in 1981 has in 2008 become the dynamic Literature, Arts & Medicine Database.

Prose and poetry pieces by physicians now appear regularly in medical journals such as the *Journal of the American Medical Association, Annals of Internal Medicine,* the *Lancet,* and *Health Affairs.* Physician narratives in the tradition of Anton Chekhov and William Carlos Williams have increased exponentially since the 1970s. Established physician-writers Richard Selzer, Jerome Groopman, Atul Gawande, Raphael Campo, Robert Coles, Jack Coulehan, Danielle Ofri, Perri Klass, Audrey Shafer, Michael LaCombe, John Stone, and David Watts have published multiple works, and many new physician-writers add their stories to fine anthologies of poetry and prose works like *On Doctoring, A Life in Medicine, Blood and Bone, Articulations,* and *Primary Care.*

And the changes in medical education that were only beginning to be made when Bergman published *The House of God* have become established. By 1998, 74 percent of U.S. medical schools taught literature and medicine, and almost 40 percent of those schools had made such study a part of a required course (Charon 23). Medical students, house officers, and practicing physicians participate in literature courses and writing workshops. Often co-taught by literary scholars and physicians, such courses appear as either required or elective components in the curriculum. Narrative accounts of patients' experiences of illness are regularly considered in medical school courses and in professional reflections on the patient-physician relationship (Charon 24). And so too are writings by physicians. The presence of courses on literature and medicine in medical humanities programs at three-fourths of medical schools in the United States has helped to create an academic place and a legitimacy for personal writing by health care profession-als. The examination of such works by physicians and medical students achieves a critical goal in medical education. It allows them to reflect on what they do in medicine and what medicine has done to them (Charon 24).

When Bergman wrote about his training experiences in 1978, he did so undercover. His pseudo-autobiography is narrated by Roy and written under a pseudonym so that Roy speaks for Sam Shem, who stands in for the authentic voice of Steve Bergman. Bergman wrote alone. For Neeta and Dagan, *Body Language* was conceived as a book not only about their stories but about the stories of a community of physicians at various stages of training in different institutions across the country.

Bergman, like Jain and Coppock, acknowledges the catharsis of writing. According to Aristotle in *Poetics,* catharsis brings about a restoration of health through the release of overwhelming emotion of great sorrow or fear or even laughter. Writing is restorative. As physician-writer Kate Scannell remarked, "writing and speaking about doctoring can save your life":

> While writing my memoir I was encouraged by Muriel Rukeyser's question: "Who will be the throat of these hours . . . Who will speak these days?" In re-sponding, I claimed my own, unique experience of being a doctor—no more or less important than a dozen disparate others', but one belonging to the whole. As each of us narrates the experiential dimensions of doctoring that only we can know, each of us uniquely becomes "the throat of the hours," speaking and writing to articulate our very lives, finding our own "continuous thread of revelation." As individuals, when we say, "This, but not that, is what I think and feel," or, "This, but not that, is who I am," we widen the truth about who we are as a group. (Scannell 781)

In 2008, the poems in *Body Language* return to *The House of God* and the medical training experience and affirm with Bergman that "the healing es-sence of narrative is not in the 'I' or the 'you' but in the 'we'" (Shem, "Fiction as Resistance" 936).

NOTES

1. Two of the members were medical school deans: Edmund Pellegrino, who had been dean at Kentucky, Tennessee, and Yale, and president of Catholic University; and George T. Harrell, who had founded the Penn State medical school two years earlier. Other members included Sam Banks, at what was then the Health Center of the University of Florida; Ronald McNeur, at the University of California San Francisco Medical School; and E. A. Vastyan, at the University of Texas Medical Branch at Galveston Texas Branch. Banks and Vastyan had both studied literature. In addition to theologians and physicians, literary scholars and social scientists joined the dialogue between the disciplines of literature and medicine (see Trautmann).

2. It was human care in medical education that C. P. Snow thought had been compromised by the predominance of scientific knowledge. He suggested that proper medical training would include the critical reading of novels as one obvious way to bridge the gap between the art and science of health care. George Engel's new model for medical education, which appeared in the journal *Science* at the same time as Snow's article in the *Journal of the American Medical Association,* suggested a new approach to the patient that would give the biomedical dimensions of the patient's disease and the patient as person equal attention.

WORKS CITED

Bruer, John T., and K. S. Warren. "Liberal Arts and the Premedical Curriculum." *Journal of the American Medical Association* 245 (1981): 364–66.

Charon, Rita. "Literature and Medicine: Origins and Destinies." *Academic Medicine* 75.1 (2000): 23–27.

Engel, George. "The Need for a New Medical Model: A Challenge for Biomedicine." *Science* 196 (1977): 129–36.

Frank, Arthur W. *Wounded Storyteller: Body, Illness, and Ethics.* Chicago: University of Chicago Press, 1995.

Graham, Peter W. "Recent Works of Interest." *Literature and Medicine* 1 (1982): 47–52.

Jain, Neeta, Dagan Coppock, and Stephanie Brown Clark, eds. *Body Language: Poems of the Medical Training Experience.* New York: BOA Editions, 2006.

Jones, Anne Hudson. "Images of Physicians in Literature: Medical Bildingsromans." *Lancet* 348 (1996): 734–36.

Marston, Wendy. "Medicine's Steamy Side, for and about Interns." *New York Times* 6 July 1999.

Pellegrino, Edmund. "Medical Humanism and Technologic Anxiety." *The Role of the Humanities in Medical Education.* Ed. Donnie J. Self. Norfolk, Va.: Bio-ethics Program, Eastern Virginia Medical School, 1978. 1–7.

Sawyer, A. "Wordsworth Books: Interview with author Samuel Shem." Paper copy of article from http://webseitz.fluxent.com/wiki/samuelshem. BITU Productions, 1997.

Scannell, Kate. "Writing for Our Lives: Physician Narratives and Medical Practice." *Annals of Internal Medicine* 137.9 (2002): 779–81.

Shem, Samuel. "Fiction as Resistance." *Annals of Internal Medicine* 137.11 (2002): 934–37.

Snow, C. P. "Human Care." *Journal of the American Medical Association* 225 (1973): 617–21.

Trautmann, Joanne. "Can We Resurrect Apollo?" *Literature and Medicine* 1 (1982): 1–17.

Wear, Delese. "The House of God: Another Look." *Academic Medicine* 77 (2002): 496–501.

The Popocatepetl of Medicine

ARKO ODERWALD

INTRODUCTION

Written in 1997, *Mount Misery* is the third novel of Samuel Shem. *Mount Misery* can be seen as the follow-up to *The House of God*. However, this novel never achieved the popularity of Shem's first born, at least in the Netherlands, where I live and work. So when I was reading *Mount Misery* again, my main question was, Why didn't it get the same reception as *The House of God*?

Rereading a novel is always a surprising enterprise. The reader is older and wiser (he hopes) and may have changed perspectives in the meantime. After my first reading of *Mount Misery*, for instance, I had published in 2003 a book about psychiatry and literature, which broadened my knowledge about the subject. Rereading *Mount Misery* led me to make two strong associations with literary works, which will play an important role in this essay.

DR. BECAMARTE

Joachim Maria Machado de Assis, a Brazilian writer, wrote in 1882 a short story called "The Alienist." Dr. Bacamarte is the most famous doctor in Brazil. He lives in Itaguai. Mental health in Itaguai is not really a problem. Dangerous patients are locked up in a bedroom in their homes until they die; those who are not dangerous may walk around in the streets. Becamarte, however, thinks that a mental institution is needed. He convinces the city council, gets funding, and after some time opens the Green House, the town's first mental institution. Soon it is too small for all the patients who need treatment. Becamarte is shocked by the great number of patients and comes to believe that many more people are insane than he could have imagined. The doctor begins to find more and more people imbalanced, and they are all forced to live in the Green House. The Green House allows him to develop a rational classification of madness. He distinguishes between two main categories—the dangerous and the quiet insane—and then come several subcategories, like with or without hallucinations, and the like.

The people of Itaguai protest more and more against the doctor's practices, but the rebellion is undermined by the admission of the most important members of the protesters to the hospital. Now 80 percent of the population of Itaguai is staying in the Green House. All these people are diagnosed as imbalanced and irrational.

Then Becamarte realizes what these numbers mean. Being insane is normal; being sane and rational is, on the contrary, not normal. All the patients are released, and thorough investigations demonstrate to Bacamarte that the remaining 20 percent of the people are less rational than he thought. Finally he admits himself to his own hospital, where he is the only patient.

Reading *Mount Misery* again made me think of this story. There are many similar topics in Samuel Shem's novel, which was written almost one hundred years after the story of Machado de Assis. Take, for instance, the relativity of psychiatric diagnoses or the idea that psychiatrists are, in fact, insane themselves, while some patients, in fact, are fully normal (known as Edgar Allan Poe's Dr. Tarr and Professor Fether hypothesis).

But first let me refresh your memory a little. Samuel Shem described in *The House of God* a year of residency in internal medicine. His hero is Roy Basch. In *Mount Misery*, the story of Roy Basch continues with his first-year residency in psychiatry. Between those two years Roy and Berry, his girlfriend, travel for a year around the world. So the book is situated one year after *The House of God* but was written almost twenty years after the first book. Thus, on one hand, it is situated in 10 B.P. (before Prozac), and on the other hand also in 10 A.P. Prozac, and the whole of biological psychiatry is present in the book, but so is a very strong Freudian tendency belonging much more to the time before Prozac.

Roy arrives at the mental institution called Mount Misery, where he meets his fellow residents and starts a tour through the different departments. Freudians from B.P. and a biologist from A.P. and almost every other congregation psychiatry has to offer are described in the book. The psychiatrists are in general suitable for a long stay in their own institution, much as Dr. Becamarte is in the end the only inhabitant of the Green House. There are maybe two exceptions to this rule: the head supervisor, Ike White (who commits suicide shortly after Roy starts at Mount Misery), and an almost-blind psychiatrist, Geneva Hooevens. She seems to be the only generalist in the story, combining the philosophies of all the different congregations. She is like Tiresias, the blind advisor of Oedipus, also living more or less outside the power structures of the institution.

The residents (Henry, Hannah, Win, and Arnie) are very vulnerable. Henry and Hannah stop their residency during the first year. Win and Arnie identify almost completely with their superiors and stay. One resident in his third year, Leonard Malik, is resisting the system. He is the Fat Man of this book (funny enough, very skinny, and always emphasizing the importance of sport). But he is a recovering alcoholic and has a relapse at the end of the year. Roy is also disoriented during this year. He starts an affair with another woman; he starts taking pills and drinking. His father dies, which deepens his existential crisis.

The patients, on the other hand, seem to be at the wrong place all the time. Psychiatry makes them sicker; they are quite normal without psychiatric treatment. Their stay in the institution is more or less determined by the fact that they have very good health insurance and the right diagnosis, which is heavily influenced by the same insurance. The right diagnosis is always the diagnosis the insurance pays for. There are, however, also patients in the state institution, close to Mount Misery. Their situation is horrifying, without any hope for improvement or a more dignified life. They are the real psychiatric patients, and nobody pays attention to them. The patients in Mount Misery, however, suffer from an unhealthy attractiveness to psychiatrists; sexual abuse of patients is one of the leading themes of the novel.

Mount Misery, which is built on a hill, is composed of several buildings. It is a classical psychiatric hospital of the end of the nineteenth century: surrounded by lots of trees, a quiet place in the countryside where the mind can rest. On the top of the hill are two buildings called Heidelberg east (addiction) and west (psychopharmacology), which are separated from each other by a canyon and connected by a bridge. The buildings are replicas of the city towers in Heidelberg.

This very short description of the novel tries to give the impression of hyperbole, for that is indeed what *Mount Misery* is. This becomes clear when we compare this book with another description of becoming a psychiatrist. Robert Klitzman's book *In the House of Dreams and Glass,* for instance, published in 1995, shows lots of similarities with *Mount Misery* but is presented as nonfiction and lacks the hyperbolic dimension of Mount Misery. Difference in style is, of course, a general difference between an autobiographical account, which Klitzman's book is, and a novel, like *Mount Misery,* even when the novel is rooted in the biography of the writer.

The hyperbolic nature of *Mount Misery* is not really surprising in the case of Samuel Shem. *The House of God* is written in the same way. But interestingly enough, *The House of God* seems to be much more appreciated and, surprisingly for a novel, more commonly seen as the reality of medicine than *Mount Misery* is.

In the Netherlands, almost every medical student reads *The House of God* when he or she is in the last two clinical years before becoming a doctor. And many of them talk about that book in terms of recognition: this is what hospital medicine is like. But, as I have pointed out, this seems not to be the case with *Mount Misery. Mount Misery* has not become the standard novel that tells what it is to become a psychiatrist. One of the reasons why it may not be seen as the standard book is its exaggeration, which is the result of the author's hyperbolic style. But that is (most of the time) not used as an argument against what is seen as the realism of *The House of God*. Above all, the comparison with Klitzman's book, reflecting the reality, shows the similarities with what we may call the reality of psychiatry. So why is the hyperbolic style regarded as a flaw in *Mount Misery* but not in *The House of God*?

UNDER THE VOLCANO

Before I try to formulate a possible answer to this question, I would like to share with you another association I had when rereading *Mount Misery*. The description of Mount Misery itself made me think of the description of the town Quauhnahuac, the Mexican city where Geoffrey Firmin, the protagonist of *Under the Volcano* by Malcolm Lowry, lives. A *barranco*, or canyon, splits the town in two (Geoffrey will die in it), and a volcano, Popocatepetl, is an ever-present threat to the town. After having this association, I also reread *Under the Volcano* to see if I could find more interesting similarities than just this image of mountains and canyons. It is very obvious that *Under the Volcano* is about an alcoholic man. And since we know that Malcolm Lowry was an alcoholic himself, we are very much inclined to think of this as a novel about addiction. Geoffrey Firmin is an alcoholic consul in the town of Quauhnahuac in Mexico. The day is the Day of the Dead, November 1. On this day, his wife, Yvonne, returns to Geoffrey. She left him because of his addiction, but Yvonne also has slept with both his best friend, Jacques, and his half-brother, Hugh. Geoffrey begged her to return, but now that she is back, it seems to be impossible for him to reaffirm their love. Instead, the novel describes this one day with Geoffrey, Hugh, and Yvonne that leads to the death of the two lovers, Geoffrey and Yvonne.

But there is much more in this novel than the psychological drama of an alcoholic. In chapter 8, for instance, there is a description of a bus trip. The bus stops because there is a dying Indian beside the road. Geoffrey and Hugh get off the bus, but they don't help the Indian. The Mexican police may come any moment, and Geoffrey and Hugh may be involved in a murder. Nobody helps the Indian. Back in the bus, they see that the man in front of them counts the money he has taken from the Indian. Blood is on his hands. The Indian is a courier carrying money for the peasants who had received land taken from the original landowners. He was probably attacked by the militia of the landowners or their accomplices, the Fascists.

This is the political dimension in *Under the Volcano*, but even more prominent is a strong moral dimension with universal tendencies. Geoffrey is guilty of not helping his fellow man, guilty of rejecting the real world, and guilty of withdrawing into his alcoholic world. That is why he has to die. Geoffrey dies by order of the chief of the Fascists, whom he encounters in the Farolito café, a (literally and symbolically) hellish place. The chief of the Fascists is also the *jefe de jardineros*, chief of the gardeners. This is no coincidence. In a very long letter of January 2, 1946, to his publisher Jonathan Cape, Lowry wrote of his book: "This novel is concerned principally with the forces in man which cause him to be terrified of himself. It is also concerned with the guilt of man, with his remorse, with his ceaseless struggling toward the light under the weight of the past, and with his doom. The allegory is that of the Garden of Eden" (*Selected Letters* 66).

So we have started to read a novel about alcoholism and end in an allegory about hell and paradise. The connection between the two is the moral concept of humanity. I think this is also the case in *Mount Misery*. You start to read about a guy who becomes a psychiatrist, and you get a psychological perspective on him and his colleagues. At first it is a bildungsroman, like *The Magic Mountain*. But then it becomes more and more a political novel about psychiatry and a moral novel about humanity in psychiatry. Yet *Mount Misery* is not really perceived in this way. The elements of this transformation are also present in *The House of God*. So we have not found our answer to the question yet.

BECOMING A DOCTOR

My father was a urologist. When I left high school and wondered what I would like to study, he advised medicine for two reasons: "If you don't know what you want right now, medicine is the ideal field of study to postpone your choice for minimal six years" and "Time makes all medical students physicians."

The first four preclinical years in the Netherlands are relatively easy. An average intellect, an ability to learn all kinds of big and little facts, and discipline get you there. In the last two clinical years, when you try several disciplines for a few weeks, everybody seems to judge you in a particular way when you are not that brilliant and do not have a gift for a particular discipline. For instance, the neurologist says, "As long as you do not become a neurologist, you may pass." They all say that you may pass as long as you do not say what your plans are. Of course, they will stop you if you really are not prepared to be a doctor, but this has been the case surprisingly seldom in the last two years. In other words, in the period that is dealt with in *The House of God,* both the readers and the heroes of the book are only more or less passing by; they are tourists. Their present work is not necessarily their work for the rest of their lives; there is no absolute need for a strong personal identification with the work that is described.

Maybe the reason why *The House of God* is such a success, even now and even in the Netherlands, is because it is not perceived as a political novel or a tragedy or a drama or a moral tale, but as a comedy with elements of truth. As I am writing this essay, there is in the Netherlands a television series about a medical student in the hospital. It is based on a novel that has already sold 60,000 copies (this is a lot in my little country). It was written under a pseudonym by a former student at my university. The novel is based on her own experience as a medical student. Reading this novel, I am surprised how little has changed in medicine since *The House of God,* considering the fact that hundreds of hours in communication skills and medical humanities have been added to the curriculum since then. But even more surprising is that nobody seems to notice that almost nothing has changed (even the necessity of writing such a book under a pseudonym). The general attitude seems to be that this is what medicine is, with a funny touch, of course. It does not, for instance, give rise to feelings of shame about the way doctors treat their patients. There does not seem to be a general message to be understood or a general lesson to be learned. In *The House of God,* the hyperbolic witty style also allows the author to hide the meaning.

For me this offers a possible explanation why *Mount Misery* never attained the same status as *The House of God.* The readers of *Mount Misery* who have a medical background are psychiatrists or they are not. If not, a probable reaction is "Typical psychiatry." If you are a psychiatrist, the reaction is probably "But this is not the reality" or "But I am a different kind of psychiatrist." The novel is more specific; therefore for some it is too distant from their experience, for others too close. However, Roy Basch (and the narrator of *Mount Misery,* who is at the time of writing a psychiatrist himself) is also a different person than the Roy in *The House of God.* In *Mount Misery* he is not passing by anymore; psychiatry is his future life. His identification with the subject is stronger; the message about psychiatry is therefore more powerful. Even if the ground patterns of both books are similar, the hyperbole in *Mount Misery* is more overexaggerated. The hyperbolic style is more pronounced and does not hide the meaning enough. Patients and doctors are stronger adversaries than in *The House of God;* this culminates in the central theme of the book: the sexual abuse of patients by doctors, which causes several suicides. This is clearly not funny anymore, but it is also not hyperbolic anymore. The fact that *Mount Misery* has a plot makes it more difficult to connect the hyperbolic style only to wittiness.

I realize that the implication of my argument is that if you write a good hyperbolic novel like *The House of God,* the readers may not catch the meaning hidden in the hyperbole, whereas if you contaminate your hyperbole with cruel reality and the meaning is clear, there is a chance it will be rejected by readers.

But that is all in the game of writing a novel. The reality is that the plot in an action-driven story might distract the reader from deeper, symbolic meanings. Unfortunately, novels have readers, just as hospitals have patients. Nevertheless, in my opinion, *Mount Misery* is still worthwhile reading for several reasons connected to the special position psychiatry has in medicine.

THE POPOCATEPETL OF MEDICINE

As in *Under the Volcano,* humanity is the key to understanding *Mount Misery.* People have the moral obligation to help each other. Leonard Malik is the personification of this principle, but he stands almost alone. As for the rest, everybody on the doctors' side seems to be busy trying to reach the top of the mountain: world fame. Patients are a means to get to the top. "Patients are certainly not there to be cared for," say the biologists. "You should never believe them," say the psychoanalysts. Although the first law of Mount Misery is that there are no laws in psychiatry, this is not the opinion of the doctors of Mount Misery. According to them, there are strong laws, although one group thinks the laws are psychoanalytic, and another group thinks they are biological. In practice these laws are flexible enough to explain every patient in a way that favors the personal goals of the physicians.

As it was in the story of Machado de Assis, the theoretical flexibility or weakness of psychiatry is certainly still part of psychiatry, even today. There is still a minute difference between normal and abnormal, sane and insane. And patients' problems are most of the time chronic and not easy to cure. Therefore, caring still is (or should be) an important concept in modern psychiatry. In this way the psychiatrist can change the pathological suffering into normal suffering, as Freud said.

But in *Mount Misery* it seems that humanity and science are sworn enemies, that empathy and the medical gaze are mutually exclusive. The medical gaze (and power) wins at first. The empathetic Malik relapses in his addiction. Hannah and Henry give up the training. Roy becomes addicted. Then empathy wins when the sexual abuse of patients is revealed. But it is not a real victory; the real victory would be an integration of empathy and the medical gaze. They can be enemies, but they can also be friends. The struggle between them is perhaps bigger in psychiatry than in somatic medicine. For instance, in psychiatry more patients have to be convinced that they have a problem than do patients in somatic medicine. The use of force based on the principle of humanity is more common. William Carlos Williams has shown us how difficult the combination of the two is. In psychiatry this is part of the job.

The theoretical flexibility, the greater need for care and fewer possibilities of a cure, the social impact of a psychiatric disease, more patients who are not convinced that they have a disease (and the dangers connected to this disease), the force that is sometimes needed—these are elements that make the practice of psychiatry different from the practice of somatic medicine, as described in *The House of God*. Psychiatric patients also need more humanity, more social support, and more political advocacy than most somatic patients. So when you are on the top of the mountain called psychiatry, it may well turn out to be a volcano. Psychiatry is the Popocatepetl, not the Magic Mountain, of medicine. That is what *Mount Misery* tells us.

WORKS CITED

Klitzman, Robert. *In a House of Dreams and Glass: Becoming a Psychiatrist.* New York: Simon and Schuster, 1995.
Lowry, Malcolm. *Selected Letters.* London: Jonathan Cape, 1967.
———. *Under the Volcano.* New York: Reynal and Hitchcock, 1947.
Machado de Assis, Joachim Maria. *The Psychiatrist and Other Stories.* Berkeley and Los Angeles: University of California Press, 1963.
Shem, Samuel. *The House of God.* New York: St. Martin's Press, 1978.
———. *Mount Misery.* New York: Fawcett Columbine, 1997.

*Women's Perspectives
and Criticism*

Objects, Not Allies: Nurses in The House of God and Graduate Medical Education

AMY HADDAD

I graduated from a bachelor's degree nursing program in 1975. For the first four months after graduation, I worked on a general medical/surgical unit at a teaching hospital. I wore a white uniform—a pants suit, as I recall, since dresses were difficult to work in—and no cap. I ditched my unwieldy cap as soon as I graduated. I changed to street clothes when I moved to a new position in psychiatry on the adolescent unit. By the time I read *The House of God* in 1978, I was working as the head nurse on the locked adult intensive care unit in psychiatry. I remember reading the book but only in general terms. I do remember being somewhat amused that the interns were so shocked by the human messiness they encountered and surprised at the depth of their struggle to survive the year at the House of God. I wondered what the interns thought they were getting into when they entered medicine. As nursing students, we didn't pay much attention to how the medical students were educated and had no interaction with them in our classes or clinical work. We knew they started with cadavers and we started with each other and real patients. I am certain we had a much better idea of what to expect when we became real nurses, as we learned firsthand what it was like to be on the receiving end of care. Our education began with experiences that established mutuality with our patients. We started intravenous lines on each other, practiced giving injections, endured novice attempts at inserting nasogastric tubes, and even gave each other baths. This kind of introduction to caregiving makes an indelible impression that sustains a kindred spirit with patients. It becomes a habit of the heart to think, "I, or someone I love, could be on the receiving end of this." You cannot be brought to your knees by the suffering and horror you see in clinical practice if you are already kneeling.

Some things that did stay with me from my first reading of *The House of God* were acronyms such as "gomer" and "LOL in NAD," but I don't know if I recall it from my initial reading of the book or the fact that "gomer" and other language from *The House of God* made their way into health care lexicon and popular culture.

Thinking back to my first reading, I don't remember anything about the portrayal of nurses or the numerous sexual escapades described in the book.

Perhaps this was because my own experiences were so dramatically different from those described in the book. Sexual encounters were rare at the hospital where I worked, as far as I knew. No liaisons occurred in closets or the isolation rooms where we put patients in restraints. Granted, we didn't deal with death on a daily basis in psychiatry, but the work was challenging nonetheless. I only encountered a handful of residents and interns in psychiatry. Those encounters were uneventful. However, interactions with attending physicians in both the medical/surgical area and psychiatry were laced with discrimination and verbal and physical abuse. I was yelled at and called obscene names when I made the mistake of bothering a physician at home to clarify an order or report a change in patient status. I was jabbed in the chest on several different occasions and had objects like charts and pitchers thrown at me in anger.

Rereading the book, I don't see how I could have missed the way nurses are characterized in *The House of God*. Clearly, something has changed in the thirty years since I first read the book. Of course I have changed. I am older, more aware of sexism and stereotypes about nurses, more skilled in working the patriarchal system in health care, and certainly less tolerant of spending wasted time and energy to overcome the barriers to fulfill nursing's potential. What also changed is my focus as I read the book. This time, my emotional response was one of anger and disgust as I specifically looked for the places in the text where nurses were mentioned (more than seventy times) and how nurses were portrayed. I set out to see how the intern-nurse relationship was described, because I believe that nurses have an important but perhaps hidden and unappreciated role in graduate medical education. I thought that a collegial relationship among nurses and interns and residents could be one of the remedies to the isolation and loneliness of the intern's experience. Also, I think that nurses have a lot to teach new physicians. I wondered if the relationship between nurses and physicians had changed. Are we more likely to be colleagues or allies in health care today than the physicians and nurses in the book?

Comparing and contrasting the intern-nurse relationship as depicted in *The House of God* with contemporary nurse-physician relationships turned out to be almost impossible since the relationships in *The House of God* are so distorted. But perhaps that is the point, since the book is satiric. Shem does not categorize the book as satire and has maintained that "the events found in *The House of God* really happened—even the most horrific of them, the Black Crow Award given to the intern requesting the most postmortems" (Wear 498). Still, Shem uses the techniques of satire such as exaggeration, incongruity, and parody. So, I wasn't sure if my anger was appropriately placed. I could be mad about the characterization of nurses, but was I missing the point? Was Shem making fun of the social conditions that shape nursing's role in health care or just making fun of nurses? I had to think long and hard about how seriously I was to take the portrayal of the nurse characters in the book. If every character is fair game and open to ridicule and exaggeration, is it right for me to take offense at the outrageous stereotypes of the nurses in *The House of God*? I think that even though Shem exaggerates the character traits and failings of his fellow interns, there are also positive traits and a kind of nobility attributed to several characters, such as the policemen, Berry, and especially the Fat Man. Sympathy is solicited for the interns. Readers are drawn into the outrage expressed by the interns regarding the way they are treated. We share their grief when Potts commits suicide. Even a reader who doesn't know a thing about graduate medical education would come away from the book with the conviction that this is not the way interns should be taught. So, I think it is fair to ask the question: Is this the way nurses should be treated? Further, does Shem even consider the objectification of nurses a social condition that needs to be changed? I would argue that Shem is not interested in drawing attention to the subservient role of nurses in health care. Nurses in *The House of God* are at best part of the background, and at worst idiotic, incompetent sex objects.

There is no sympathy for the nurse characters in *The House of God*. They are peripheral to the anguish of the residents, even peripheral to the patients, although nurses are mentioned in proportion to their true numbers in clinical practice. However, they are generally portrayed as submissive, weak, and ineffectual. Their roles are stereotypically defined, and the most appealing characters are cute, sexy, and dumb. Nurses' concerns seem to have little to do with patient care and a great deal to do with fulfilling male fantasies. Their relationships with other nurses are thinly described or ludicrous, as in the orgy scene. Few of the nurses in *The House of God* are developed characters. Most are coarsely drawn fantasies that serve as the outlets, or perhaps repositories, for the frustration, doubt, anger, and guilt of the interns. Sexual fantasies are a major device used by Shem to allow the interns, such as the narrator, Roy Basch, "to cope with anxiety or frustration by allowing him to mentally create a relationship where none exists, to act out in his imagination sexual or aggressive behaviors that are forbidden in reality or to transform a person or relationship into whatever is desired. Fantasies are not accidents; they are representations of unconscious conflicts and wishes. Fantasies beget myths" (Muff 114). Myths give rise to stereotypes.

THE CHARACTERIZATION OF NURSES IN *THE HOUSE OF GOD*

Stereotypes of nurses play at the edge of the real drama in *The House of God* as the interns struggle to maintain their humanity in the face of incredible pressure. Not surprisingly, these stereotypes are derived from those about women in general but are heightened because of the intimate nature of nursing. Unfortunately, the following selected stereotypes about nurses still appear in the media today. All of them are evident in *The House of God*.

- Nurse as Ministering Angel—the altruistic, gentle, non-human healer
- Nurse as Handmaiden or Servant to the Physician—follows orders without question
- Nurse as Sex Symbol—seductive temptress
- Nurse as Fluff Ball—the nursing version of the dumb blonde stereotype
- Nurse as Old Maid or Battle-Ax—rigid, cold, and mean (Muff 120)

Sometimes several of these stereotypes are used to refer to the same character in the same sentence. Roy Basch describes one of the nurses as a "voracious nurse named Angel—Angel, who never ever did, the whole long year, to anyone's knowledge, string together a complete sentence made of real words" (Shem 4). Here we have the ministering, aptly named, Angel (although she is not really ministering to the patients but to the interns), who is a sex symbol and a fluff ball—someone who is so stupid that she can't complete a sentence. How did she get through nursing school? It must follow that it doesn't take brains to be a nurse.

Nurses are clearly subservient to physicians in *The House of God*: "When a BMS doctor tells a BMS nurse to do something, you can be sure it will be done, and it will be done right" (17). There are only a few direct examples of this particular stereotype of nurse as handmaiden, but it is clear that nurses only act on a physician's orders and make very few decisions on their own. Most of the actual nursing activity described in the book involves asking the physician for orders or clarification of the obvious.

The sex symbol stereotype is without question the most common one in the book. Nurses are described in terms that border on the pornographic. These few examples tell the story of the nurse acting as seductress while performing the most banal activities:

> I saw Molly, perky transparent Molly, bending over the bed, fiddling with the sheet. She kept her legs straight, so her miniskirt rode up her thighs, and with a final reach over to the far side of the bed, she hiked the hem up over her ass, showering me with the rainbow-and-flower pattern of her little-girl panties, snug against the firm full glutei folds that formed an awning over the juicy female thing that grew up there. I could feel a half-chub mumbling and squirming in my whites. (56)

The nurses in *The House of God* are treated as sex objects and, on the whole, don't seem to resent it. In fact, they are promiscuous and active, willing participants in everything from intercourse in the on-call room to group sex. Patient care doesn't seem to be on anyone's mind as the nurses attend to the sexual needs of the overburdened interns.

> With Molly, so far, there had been no talk, there'd been only the straight bendovers, the clefts and the round full hollows, the red nails and blue lids and panties splashed with flowers and rainbows, and the laughter amidst the gomers and the dead. Molly was the promise of a breast against an arm. Molly was recess. (64)

> At eleven came the striptease, the nursing change of shift: smooth leading thighs, a black lace panty rolling down as the tight dungarees came off, flashing pubic hair, the side slope of a jiggly breast, the full frontal of two firm ones, errant nipples, the works. (305)

Sexual teasing is not accidental; it is purposeful. According to the Fat Man, "That nursing maneuver, where they bend from the waist and flash their ass. Called the Straight Bendover Nursing Maneuver. Learn it in nursing school" (57). The striptease and other maneuvers seem to be about the only thing nurses learned in school, because the House of God is plagued by nurses who are so incompetent that they harm and kill patients.

The stereotype of the fluff ball or dumb nurse is a dim second to the nurse as seductress (no pun intended) in *The House of God*. One nurse is so stupid that she can't read a sphygmomanometer:

> The nurse said there was a man I'd better see right away, his blood pressure being "patent pending over 150."
>   "Patent pending over 150? What the hell's that?"
>   "At the top of the scale where the mercury ends, the machine says patent pending. The highest it goes." (197)

Another doesn't know what to do when a patient has a life-threatening arrhythmia: "Early in the morning I was awakened by the nurse saying that Harry was in a crazy cardiac rhythm and having a chest pain and looking like he was dying and should she call a cardiac arrest?" (264). Even in 1978, nurses knew what to do when a patient was in cardiac arrest, and it wasn't to go to the on-call room and wake up the intern. Nurses are not only dumb; they are downright dangerous to patients and the interns. As one of the interns, Runt, tells the other interns about an exchange transfusion on a patient referred to as "the Yellow Man": "I'd taken a needle out of the groin and was about to put it into the last bag of blood, and that porpoise, Celia the nurse, well, she held up this other needle from the

Yellow Man's belly and . . . stuck it in my hand" (67). The Runt then worries for most of the rest of the book that he will die from the same disease that has afflicted the Yellow Man. Then there is the nurse whose neglect kills a patient: "Tina had died by being inadvertently murdered by a nurse in dialysis who'd mixed up the bottles. Instead of diluting Fast Tina's blood, the machine had concentrated it further, and all the water had been pulled out of Tina's body and her brain had shrunk and rattled around in her skull like a pea while the nurse sat and read Cosmopolitan" (255). Of course she would be reading *Cosmopolitan* while she ignores a dying patient. This triple slam (incompetent, uncaring, and a Cosmo girl) is particularly insulting and indicative of the lack of knowledge of the real roles and responsibilities of nurses.

The battle-ax nurse is present in *The House of God* but infrequently mentioned. She is someone to be feared, as in this description of Dini, the charge nurse in the emergency room:

> Dini took me and Elihu on a tour of the premises. Although she was attractive, there was something disturbing about her. What was it? Her eyes. Her eyes were hard blank disks showing nothing in back of them. She had worked this beachhead for twelve years. She showed us the different rooms: gynecology, surgery, medicine, and then, last, room 116, which she affectionately called "The Grenade Room." (173)

Dini's physical attributes are described first so that we understand that her appearance doesn't contribute to her battle-ax status. Yet she is disturbing and has blank, dead eyes. The interns are scared of her. When she tells them to do something, they do it. If the battle-ax nurse isn't frightening and attractive, the interns treat her with derision:

> "Salli and Bonni—they both wear caps and tin nursing-school badges like meter maids—who say things to the gomers like 'Now we eat our custard, sport.' The worst" (121). "We antagonized Salli and Bonni for stopping Eddie's TURF of the Lady of Lice—he'd neglected to put down on her three-part placement form who would meet her in St. Louis—mentioning in passing the word 'cunts,' which sent both of them and our female BMS flying out of the room." (277)

The strongest message delivered by all these stereotypes is that nurses play a marginal role in the care of patients. The few examples of actual nursing practice that are included are oversimplified. We see that nurses provide basic care to patients:

Just before I left I wanted to say good-bye to Molly. I found her carrying a bedpan toward the disposal. I walked with her, the shit sloshing in the pan, and said, "It's not a very romantic way to meet someone." (54)

Nurses also report problems to the interns and physicians, never providing a solution, and passively wait for directions:

The nurse came in and said, "Mr. Lazarus has just had a bowel movement that is all blood."

"Hey, that's really funny, Maxine. You got a great sense of humor."

"No, I'm serious. The bed is solid blood." (121)

The one description of nursing care in the whole book that comes closest to actual practice is in the scene dealing with the terminally ill patient, Dr. Sanders: "I watched Molly take care to clip his fingernails and toenails so he wouldn't scratch himself and bleed or get infected. I watched everyone keep sterile around his bed" (156). The nurse is rendering personal care and she does "take care" to be gentle with this dying patient. However, the action in question requires minimal skill. Anyone can clip nails, so it still doesn't provide an accurate representation of what nurses know and can contribute to patient care. Thus, the characterizations of nurses in *The House of God* and their relationships with physicians are plagued with stereotypes and therefore lack the foundation upon which to build a true working relationship.

CONTEMPORARY NURSE-PHYSICIAN RELATIONSHIPS AND GRADUATE MEDICAL EDUCATION

Considerable progress has been made in the nurse-physician relationship since the 1970s, but there is still work to be done. I refer the reader to Corser's excellent overview of the research on the contemporary nurse-physician relationship, including fundamental differences in practice and ideologies, and the inherent power differential in nursing and medicine. One way to look at the status of the nurse-physician relationship is to study places that foster positive relationships. For example, Magnet hospitals, those that have met criteria for accreditation by the American Nurses Credentialing Center, consistently report that they have "good" nurse-physician relationships. When nurses who work at Magnet hospitals are asked what characterizes a good nurse-physician relationship, they uniformly respond: good communication, mutual respect, and concern for patients (Kramer and Schmalenberg). Good communication between nurses and physicians is still a challenge because there is little interaction between nursing students and medical students during their educational programs. Therefore, they don't get a chance to practice cross-disciplinary communication until they are on the job. Opportunities for sharing in planning, making decisions, solving problems, and assuming responsibility together should be part of entry-level education in both nursing and medicine (Wilkinson and Hite).

Imbalances of power are still problematic in nurse-physician relationships. Power differentials lead to difficulties with mutual respect. The American Nurses Association Commission on Workplace Advocacy Work Group on Nurse-Physician Relationships chairperson, Donna Warzynski, notes that there "seems to be a lack of courtesy and respect for nurses' expertise and knowledge. For example, if a nurse tries to clarify or determine the rationale for an order, he or she risks being taken to task for it or gets demeaning comments, like 'How would you know that?' or 'I can have your job'" (qtd. in Trossman 65). In order to change disrespectful behavior, hospitals have to make changes at an institutional level by establishing policies to promote respect and oversight groups to deal with disruptive behavior. For example, in its 2002 alert about the nursing shortage, the Joint Commission on the Accreditation of Health Care Organizations raised the issue of the impact of nurse-physician relationships and called for a voluntary policy of zero tolerance in the workplace for verbal and other types of abuse by physicians (12).

The ideal nurse-physician relationship is a collegial one—"the essential ingredient in these relationships is equality based on 'different but equal' power and knowledge" (Kramer and Schmalenberg 36). In collegial practice, nurses and physicians know different things and both bring valuable knowledge to patient care. Knowing how the other discipline looks at the world is essential to appreciate the different skills each brings to the bedside. It appears that physicians have more work to do in this area than nurses. Journalist Suzanne Gordon noted that in interviews with nurses, "Their most common complaints were that physicians don't understand the role nurses play in the health care system, misunderstand whom nurses serve, do not value the knowledge and skill that nurses have amassed during their careers, and fail to appreciate that collaborative, cooperative, collegial relationships between physicians and nurses are central to quality patient care" (26). One distinction between physicians and nurses noted by nurse-poet Veneta Masson is particularly relevant to the ending of *The House of God*: "Whereas medicine is based on the use of tools, nursing is based on the use of self: to listen, teach, guide, support, be there. You can design, standardize, and automate tools to achieve efficacy and speed. The self, on the other hand, cannot be streamlined, packaged, or delivered. Its effective use requires time, quality time" (24).

To escape the dehumanization they encounter, most of the interns turn to psychiatry, where the essence is being with patients. Perhaps this is an area in which nurses would be particularly helpful to new physicians—to help them learn about the use of self with patients. Yet turning to nurse colleagues for help is not part of the average intern's repertoire. Changes in medical education and the behavior of medical mentors toward nurses are necessary before medical students and interns recognize nurses as allies. The type of change I am talking about is enormous; the attitudes and dramatically different ideologies are deeply entrenched. Collegial practice is still the exception, not the rule. Change of this magnitude is difficult but worth it, as there is ample evidence in the literature to support a direct link between the quality of the nurse-physician relationship and the quality of patient care (Mitchell and Shortell). Furthermore, when nurse-physician relationships are good, the work environment is characterized by less stress and strain (O'Brien-Pallas, Shamian, et al.). These two positive outcomes of collegial relationships between nurses and physicians are highly desirable in a health care system beset by errors, questionable quality, and a critical shortage of nurses.

WORKS CITED

Corser, W. "The Contemporary Nurse-Physician Relationship: Insights from Scholars outside the Two Professions." *Nursing Outlook* 48.6 (2000): 263–68.

Joint Commission on the Accreditation of Health Care Organizations. *Health Care at the Crossroads: Strategies for Addressing the Evolving Nursing Crisis.* Oakbrook Terrace, IL: Joint Commission on the Accreditation of Health Care Organizations, 2002.

Kramer, Marlene, and Claudia Schmalenberg. "Securing 'Good' Nurse-Physician Relationships." *Nurse Management* 34.7 (2003): 34–38.

Masson, Veneta. *Ninth Street Notebook—Voice of a Nurse in the City.* Washington, D.C.: Sage Femme Press, 2001.

Mitchell, Pamela, and Steven Shortell. "Adverse Outcomes and Variations in Organization of Care Delivery." *Medical Care* 35 (1997): NS19–NS32.

Muff, Janet. "Handmaiden, Battle-Ax, Whore: An Exploration into Fantasies, Myths and Stereotypes about Nurses." *Socialization, Sexism, and Stereotyping: Women's Issues in Nursing.* Ed. Janet Muff. St. Louis, MO: Mosby, 1982. 113–56.

O'Brien-Pallas, Linda, Judith Shamian, et al. "Work-Related Disability in Canadian Nurses." *Journal of Nursing Scholarship* 36.4 (2004): 352–57.

Shem, Samuel. *The House of God.* New York: Random House, 1978.

Trossman, Susan. "Professional Respect: The CWPA and Magnet Facilities Work to Improve Nurse-Physician Relationships." *American Journal of Nursing* 103.3 (2003): 65–67.

Wear, Delese. "*The House of God:* Another Look." *Academic Medicine* 77.6 (2002): 496–501.

Wilkinson, Connie S., and Kari J. Hite. "Nurse-Physician Collaborative Relationship on Nurses' Self-Perceived Job Satisfaction in Ambulatory Care." *Lippincott's Case Management* 6.2 (2001): 68–78.

"Fiction as Resistance":
The Fat Man and the Woman Reader

ANNE HUDSON JONES

> Re-vision—the act of looking back, of seeing with fresh eyes, of entering an
> old text from a new critical direction—is for us more than a chapter in cultural
> history: it is an act of survival.
>
> ADRIENNE RICH, "WHEN WE DEAD AWAKEN"

Nearly thirty years later, I still remember the first time that I read *The House of
God*. It was in the spring of 1979, not long after I arrived at the Institute for the
Medical Humanities in Galveston. Two of my new (male) colleagues urged me
to read it, assuring me that the novel would give me important and necessary
insight into the real world of contemporary clinical medicine. When I reported
back to them that I was having trouble reading it because I was offended by the
sexist (if not pornographic) opening pages, they encouraged me not to judge
the book by its first pages and its superficial sexism. I kept reading. But soon I
was also offended by the characterization of Jo, the only woman resident, who
is represented not only as a bad doctor but also as a person so cut off from normal human relationships and feelings that no one would want to identify with
her. Even the character of Berry didn't help much. Although she is wise and
forgiving, she is also out of the fray, professionally and emotionally, presumably
by choice. I couldn't help wondering, though, whether she is out of the fray
by choice or as a result of whatever combination of forces made it so difficult
for women to go to medical school at that time. Why a clinical psychologist
instead of a psychiatrist? In short, my plight was that of the woman reader of
any text that presents male experience as the norm and represents women only
as sex objects (the nurses and social workers), as rigid and obnoxious authority
figures (Jo), or as romantic interests (Berry). With whom was I to identify as
I read this novel?

Part of the magic and power (some would say the danger) of narrative fiction is its ability to direct the reader's identification with certain characters by
carefully structuring the point of view from which the events are recounted.
Thus, readers can step vicariously into the worlds of characters very unlike themselves and learn from those fictive experiences. In Kafka's *The Metamorphosis*,

for example, most readers identify with the character Gregor Samsa, who has already been transformed into an *ungeheures Ungeziefer* (usually translated as vermin or giant beetle or cockroach) by the first sentence of the tale. Having easily enough identified with Gregor when I read *The Metamorphosis,* I soon settled down as a reader of *The House of God,* accepted the first-person point of view, and began to identify with Roy Basch and his fellow male interns. I had already had years of experience identifying with male characters, after all. Thus, having quelled my initial resistance, I kept reading and discovered why my colleagues recommended the novel and why Kathryn Montgomery Hunter proclaimed, "Although it is not a great book, for the moment—particularly for doctors and teachers of doctors—it is an important one" (136).

In the years since my initial reading, I have taught the novel regularly (almost every year) to medical students and to graduate students in the medical humanities. Every time, I have had to encourage the women readers, especially the women nurses, to persevere, quell their resistance to the offensive ways that the women characters are represented, and keep reading. Year after year, I have told them that this is the author's first novel and that he may not, therefore, have realized the huge risks he took in alienating women readers so deeply that many probably would stop reading long before they could appreciate the novel's endorsement of important values of medicine and patient care. I have pointed out the author's awareness of the sexism of the novel and his inclusion of Roy Basch's regret as early as the first pages of the novel: "We had savaged the women of the House. . . . And I know now that the sex in the House of God had been sad and sick and cynical and sick, for like all our doings in the House, it had been done without love, for all of us had become deaf to the murmurs of love" (11–12). I have also pointed out the exchange in which Basch accuses the Fat Man of sounding "like a male chauvinist" because he is "saying women like Jo make lousy doctors because they're women." The Fat Man responds with surprise and insists that he is "saying women like Jo make lousy people because they are doctors, just like some men do. The profession is a disease. It doesn't care what sex you are" (106). I have underscored the Fat Man's words by pointing out that the novel has no lack of male characters who are both lousy doctors and lousy people. All of this is true. And it has usually been enough to persuade the women students in my classes to keep reading the book.

Yet even after all these years, I find my own apologetic arguments on behalf of the author unsatisfying. What still seems inexcusable is the choice of making the only woman resident in the novel both a lousy person and a lousy doctor. Jo stands out not because she is a lousy person and a lousy doctor—there are indeed many of those among the novel's male characters—but because she is the only woman resident. Maybe if there were other women residents in the cast of characters who were not lousy people and lousy doctors, it wouldn't matter so much. As it is, however, Jo becomes for the interns of the House an adversary much like Big Nurse is for McMurphy and the other male patients of her ward in Ken Kesey's *One Flew over the Cuckoo's Nest,* which was published more than a decade earlier, in 1962. In both novels, it is a woman authority figure who represents the worst of dehumanizing institutional power. And in both novels, male sexuality is the weapon of response. As Basch succinctly says, "Our trump card with Jo could always be sex" (122).

For several years, Shem maintained in conversations with me that *The House of God* is not a satire, that things really were as he reported them, and that if he were to go through the novel with me page by page, he could persuade me of this, episode by episode. In 1988, however, Shem indicated in his introduction to the tenth anniversary edition that things were a bit more complicated than that. In answer to the question "Was it really like that?" he says, "Yes, it was." But he continues: "In fact, the departures from reality were not what you'd think." He does not say what the departures from reality were, but among the specific things he says they were not is "the sexist way that women were treated in hospitals at that time" (5).

Not until his 2002 article "Fiction as Resistance," written for a feature series on Physician-Writers' Reflections on Their Work in *Annals of Internal Medicine,* does Shem speak openly of some of the departures from reality in *The House of God* and of the ways that he used fiction as resistance "to brutality and inhumanity, to isolation and disconnection" (935). He gives as an example the need to tell a patient bad news. In reality, he says, neither he nor any of the other doctors around him were willing to tell a woman patient with metastatic breast cancer that when the surgeons opened her up, they found her cancer so advanced that there was nothing more they could do to treat her. He says he thinks a nurse finally gave the patient the bad news that she was dying. In a situation in *The House of God* that is based on this incident, the Fat Man offers to tell the woman the truth about her condition, and he does so with kindness and compassion. Most surprisingly, Basch sees that the Fat Man does not just give her the news and leave; he is still in the woman's room later that night, playing cards with her, talking, and even laughing with her at something that happened during their card game. Shem reflects on his writing of the scene:

> In retrospect, this is why I wrote the scene, to resist the inhumanity toward these patients. I started with fact—my avoidance—then imagined what "should" have been done and put it in terms of the imagined Fat Man. In this way the reality of medical practice can filter into and through creative imaginations to fiction and then, in the reality of the text, serve as a guideline in understanding not

only how things are but how things should be. This is an example of how to resist the inhumanity of medical practice, through fiction. (935)

Shem also says in this same article that he "was just telling the truth, with some art. The art part was inadvertently what Wallace Stevens, echoing Chekhov, had suggested that art can at best do, 'things as they are are changed upon the blue guitar'" (935).

Artistic creativity and the moral imagination can give examples of how things should be even in a world in which they are not that way. In his use of the fictional Fat Man to resist a medical world that dehumanizes both patient and practitioner, Shem has created a character who will continue to serve as a model of the extremely competent and caring doctor that most medical students and residents want to become. Even as Basch does in the novel itself, some of them might well stop and ask themselves what the Fat Man would do in difficult technical, ethical, and emotional situations. The spirit of the Fat Man lives on these thirty years later, even if many of the abuses he was created to resist have been rectified—or so we hope—by greater attention to the ethical and emotional aspects of medical education and practice. The Fat Man represents, as Shem well understands, the best of fiction as resistance.

But what about the Fat Man and the woman reader? Can the Fat Man do for women medical students and residents—for women readers—what he does for Shem and many male readers? In the novel, Jo and the Fat Man represent opposing theories of medical care—from Jo's "I never do nothing. I'm a doctor, I deliver medical care" (Shem, *House* 102) to the Fat Man's Law XIII: "The delivery of medical care is to do as much nothing as possible" (420). Confronted by Basch with the Fat Man's philosophy, Jo responds aggressively: "The Fat Man is nuts. . . . I'm the captain of this ship, and I deliver medical care, which, for your information, means not doing nothing, but doing something. In fact, doing everything you can, see?" (102). Nor is she ever converted to the Fat Man's way. Thus, by the end of the novel, the woman reader who wants to endorse the values Shem has written the Fat Man to illustrate—superb technical competence, empathy for patients, and the spirit to resist institutionalized brutality and inhumanity—must denounce the unthinking and unemotional assault on patients that Jo represents. But for the woman reader to do this, she must become, as the feminist critic Judith Fetterley has described it, psychologically *immasculated*—that is, she must be able to think and read like a man rather than like a woman. To the extent that any woman reader is able to get past her initial resistance to the immediate sexism of this novel and begin to identify with Roy Basch, she has to immasculate herself and read as if she were male. Ironically, Jo has had to do something analogous to survive medical school and residency: she has had to immasculate herself and identify with the male medical hierarchy represented most prominently in the novel by Dr. Leggo, the chief of medicine. There are no other women there with whom to identify, as Jo is acutely aware. Thus, she adapts by adopting and enforcing Dr. Leggo's philosophy of medicine.

Many changes have taken place in residency education and medical practice during the past thirty years, changes that Shem's novel may have accelerated. But one of the most important changes during these years has taken place without the advocacy of Shem's novel—that is, the great increase in the number of women in medicine. The entering classes of some medical schools now are more than 50 percent women. It would be unthinkable for a hospital to have only one woman in an internal medicine residency today. As a result, the representation of women in *The House of God* now seems one of its most dated features. Perhaps it is no longer necessary for the woman reader to immasculate herself to read the novel. Armed with the knowledge that things do not have to be the way they were for women then, the resisting woman reader may be able to use her own creativity and moral imagination to use *The House of God* as a blue guitar on which to craft her own transformative vision of how things should be for all women in medicine—doctors, nurses, social workers, and lovers.

WORKS CITED

Fetterley, Judith. *The Resisting Reader: A Feminist Approach to American Literature.* Bloomington: Indiana University Press, 1978.

Hunter, Kathryn Montgomery. "The Satiric Image: Healers in *The House of God.*" *Literature and Medicine* 2 (1983): 135–47.

Rich, Adrienne. "When We Dead Awaken: Writing as Re-Vision." *College English* 34 (1972): 18–30.

Shem, Samuel. "Fiction as Resistance." *Annals of Internal Medicine* 137.11 (2002): 934–37.

———. *The House of God.* New York: Dell, 1988.

The Madwoman in the Attic

SUSAN ONTHANK MATES

I am talking to my friend Jo, the cardiologist. This, of course, is fiction, since I have no friend Jo, the cardiologist. Endocrinologists, psychiatrists, ob-gyns, even a surgeon; no cardiologist. But I digress.

We are at Starbucks, glancing around to see how low we have to keep our voices—smell the coffee, hear the chatter, jazz, clinking glasses, neighbors' greeting. Each time someone bursts through the door, spring brushes our cheeks and arms. Daffodils and baby strollers have come into bloom.

"Hey," I say, "I'm supposed to write something for the thirtieth anniversary of the publication of *The House of God*."

"Wanna check out Nordstrom?" Jo examines her high-heeled sandals, moving her foot back and forth to catch the view at different angles. "They've got a sale on shoes." Jo is petite; unlike me, she can wear whatever shoe fits her fancy and look terrific in it. She glances up, swinging shiny dark hair off cheekbones that will keep her in the game until she's ninety.

"You remember *The House of God*," I say. A toddler wanders up to us and stares with wide blue eyes. We smile at the boy, chat with his mother, ooh and aah over his cuteness. They move on, leaving a trail of dribbled milk. Back to business.

"Jo," I say. "That book, *The House of God*? Chock full of women, all stereotypes so old they go back to the orangutans?"

A middle-aged man steps back to avoid two teenagers and bumps into our table. "Sorry," he says. We smile. He returns to his conversation.

"*House of God,*" I say to Jo, threateningly.

Jo looks vague, wrinkles her nose, and shakes her head. "It's all just Pride, I think, though I can't really remember. Come on," she says, "I've got to get back by six." She starts to stand up. "I haven't told you about my date," she says. "He's hot." Jo is always dating two or three men at the same time, mostly younger than her, mostly buff. I, however, am still married to a man I met in high school. He's buff, too. Really. Well, buffer than I am.

"Of course you know that book," I say. "You're in it. Remember Roy Basch? The intern who drove you crazy? That's when you taught me all the Rules."

Jo and I go back to high school, too, though we weren't friends then. Friendship happened when we shared an apartment in Jamaica Plain; I was an intern at Best City Hospital and she was a resident at the House of God. That was awhile ago, 1975 to be exact. Weren't too many women doctors on the wards in those days, though there were far more of us than five years before, which was no doubt the problem.

Jo is standing, has fished in her purse for her keys, and is waving them in front of me. A silver heart dangles from them with a darling picture I've seen, up close, of her new granddaughter. Jo gives me a morose look. "Obviously, I taught you nothing," she says. "You were supposed to FORGET those Rules. Now come on."

"I could never have gotten through without you," I say, trotting to keep up with her as she strides to her silver Porsche.

She slides behind the wheel. "I had a wonderful residency," she says, emphatically. "Those were the days." She takes the dark glasses off her head and puts them on. "Though between you and me," she adds, "*all* the interns drove me crazy. Nature of the beast, you know, Rule #1."

RULE #1 MEDICAL TRAINING WAS HAZING FOR BOY GEEKS (HFBG).

"Come on Jo," I say, "this is your life we're talking about. You mean I shouldn't say anything about how you were treated? How obnoxious and lazy and passive-aggressive those boys were? Not to mention the way they used interminable yakking about sex with other girls as a way to insult and isolate you ('You're not sexy, nyah nyah nyah,' 'You don't belong in this boys' locker room, nyah nyah nyah'). Juvenilia. As if the rest of the world right down to the bacteria in their noses weren't having more interesting sex than they were."

"The trouble with you," she says, "is that you never accepted Rule #2. Why did you *think* doctors couldn't have reasonable shifts or learn to do careful sign-overs or treat patients respectfully, like nurses did?" She turns to examine my cheek. "That's where those wrinkles come from," she says. "Worry, worry, worry. You should get those spots lasered off."

"Jesus," I say, "watch the road. We're doctors. If you run over someone, we'll have to get out and do something."

RULE #2 IN HFBG THE GAUNTLET (SLEEPLESSNESS, UNDERSTAFFING, CRUELTY, DEHUMANIZATION, ETC.) IS ENTIRELY UNNECESSARY AND ANTITHETICAL TO THE TASK (TAKING CARE OF PATIENTS). IT EXISTS TO PERPETUATE GENERATIONS OF BGS PROVING THEIR MANHOOD.

"Why don't you write about the serious issues of medical education? Or raising kids?" Jo says. "Now that's something needs talking about. Hard to believe all that running around forking the toaster and slicing the phone cord grew up into a perfectly civilized math professor. Best thing that ever happened to me, Stevie, even if his father was a jerk."

I remember, suddenly, twenty years ago and the cracks in my kitchen's red linoleum floor, where I sat tethered to the telephone the evening my friend called to read me a chart because he couldn't bear to finish it alone. Oh God. Into my ear, an unfolding tragedy in the tongue of our training: assessments, exams, progress notes, fatigue, inexperience, lack of supervision. My friend was an expert testifying to a grand jury; the chart was that of a girl named Libby Zion. My friend and I were parents by then; he stopped here and there while we wept. And then we talked about telling the truth—after all, we'd been residents, become furious at and complicit in that system, too. I think: stereotypes aside, *The House of God* was a brave and important book. But there are many who can tell that story. We don't get to choose our roles, I sigh, or if we do, I never figured out how.

"My middle daughter," I say, "just opened off Broadway. *Jane Eyre*. Remember the madwoman, the wife from the past, locked in the attic? They've got her screaming and writhing in a box onstage that they wheel around, ignoring her, while they go on with the play."

"Rochester," says Jo, slowly, lovingly. "What about your older girl? The one you had when you were a fellow?"

"Delivering babies on the same ward where she was born; lives in the same apartment building and goes to the same medical school I did." I shake my head and smile. "I'm so proud. And with *those* Apgars."

"Pride—connected by an umbilical cord to Will. I bet she thinks you're a bitter LOL," Jo says. "Face it: we're dinosaurs. The residents she hates are all girls now."

"She complains about the same things I did," I say, defensively. "Besides, this is supposed to be about *The House of God*. Our generation."

"Move on," Jo says, honking her horn at the SUV in front of us. "Hope you brought an umbrella." The sky is beginning to cloud over. "Do you remember how to get to Nordstrom the back way?" She accelerates in the breakdown lane.

I cover my eyes in terror. "The fundamental issue is basic respect for other human beings," I say through my palms. "If you don't have respect for your colleagues, how can you have it for your patients?"

"Rule #3," she mutters. "What a Dement. You should go to the gym more often."

RULE #3 IN HFBG THE LIFE YOU RISK TO PROVE YOUR MANHOOD MUST NEVER BE YOUR OWN. THAT'S WHAT PATIENTS ARE FOR.

"Can we change the topic?" Jo asks, swerving in front of the SUV with a rude hand gesture. "Those Rules were like Mission Impossible instructions: they were supposed to go up in a poof of smoke. Never happened. A little amnesia makes the medicine go down."

"Wow," I say, "I just realized that's a brilliant variation on Rule #5. You didn't have to die young!"

Jo grits her teeth. "Doesn't matter," she says. "FORGET ABOUT IT. There's no Rule #4 anymore."

~~RULE #4 IN HFBG GIRLS ARE NOT ALLOWED.~~

RULE #5 DISALLOWED GIRLS (DGS) WHO ARE WAY SMARTER THAN THE BOY GEEKS (BGS) MUST ADHERE TO THE ROSALIND FRANKLIN MEMORIAL STEREOTYPE: INVISIBLE; BRILLIANT; PREFERABLY DIE YOUNG SO THE BGS CAN CALL YOU A SEXLESS, HUMORLESS GRIND AND/OR MENTALLY UNSTABLE WHILE THEY USE YOUR UNACKNOWL-EDGED WORK TO GET THE NOBEL PRIZE.

"Well," I say, "I was just a Rule #6. I guess that's why I can't forget." I peek then cover my eyes again. Sixty miles an hour is Jo's in-town baseline.

RULE #6 DGS WHO ARE JUST A BIT SMARTER THAN THE BGS MUST ADHERE TO THE GOOD-SPORT HOUSEWIFE STEREOTYPE: INVISIBLE; TALK FOOTBALL; CLEAN UP SCUT, PATIENTS, MISUNDERSTANDINGS; SAY NOTHING WHEN THE SEXUAL ATTRIBUTES OF OTHER GIRLS (NURSES) ARE DISCUSSED RIGHT IN FRONT OF YOU AS IF (1) IT WEREN'T DEMEANING TO THE NURSES AND (2) YOU HAVE NO SEXUAL ATTRIBUTES.

"The reason you can't forget," says Jo, "is that you are unfulfilled." She leans out the window to let the wind blow through her hair.

"Isn't that the point?" I shout. "We *lived* it. How many Jos ended up where they would have if they'd been boys? Dreams were crushed, careers lost, financial plans destroyed, young families stressed to the breaking point. Discrimination is never trivial, especially when it's lied about so you can't begin to predict or understand your life. I'd rather talk about medical training or the ethical questions implicit in *The House of God,* but if we who *were* those girls don't say anything, who will? Isn't that an ethical question? What about the next group who inherits the stereotypes? Asian boys already get the Rosalind Franklin Boring Grind Special. If black and Latino girls aren't lumped with Nurses-for-Sex, they're permanently stuck in Good-Sport Housewife."

Jo sees a red light and accelerates. "You'd be a hell of a lot happier," she says, "if you'd just gotten your act together and taken Rule #7 into account."

RULE #7 DGS WHO DON'T PLAY ALONG WITH THE ABOVE ARE PUNISHED WITH THE INVISIBILITY CLOAK BY BOYS ABOVE THEM IN THE HIERARCHY AND PASSIVE AGGRESSION BY THOSE BELOW.

"But it was you who taught me Rule #8," I screech.

RULE #8 DGS WHO PLAY ALONG FAIL, TOO. THAT'S WHY YOU WERE THE ONLY DG EVERY TIME YOU HOISTED YOURSELF A RUNG UP THE LADDER. HEY, STUPID, WHERE DID YOU THINK ALL THE SMART YOUNG DGS AHEAD OF YOU WENT?

"Susan, Susan," says Jo, pulling into the Nordstrom parking lot. "Take it easy. Pride is the deadliest of the Deadlies, you know. We're old ladies now. It's all about Rule #9, and you're long overdue."

RULE #9 AGE 51 = PSALM 51

"You always were more mature than me," I tell Jo. "That's why you forget so well. What's that psalm, again?" I sneeze from the tornado of pollen that's come through the open window. Thank God for the wide asphalt parking lot, unmarred by greening things.

Jo sighs. "In the Extremely New Standard Version: *It's not all about you.*"

"Is that the one with 'the bones which thou hast broken'? I can relate to that," I say, though to be honest, I am completely confused, and, besides, my nose is running and I can't find a tissue.

Jo looks ruminatively at the darkening sky. She rolls up the window. "You know the feel of your left hand on someone's shoulder," she says, "while your right holds the stethoscope and life whacks in your ear?" She slides out of the car, slams the door, and heads for Nordstrom. "An honor. A privilege. Probably we aren't worthy of it; weren't then, either."

"Yes," I say, following her. "One tends to lose track of that." It's begun to drizzle.

"Hurry up, all the good shoes will be gone."

I scurry after her as the rain begins in earnest, washing my face, saturating my body. "Is it because of Pride, that new Rule, #9?" I ask when I catch up.

She's pulled the hood up on her raincoat. She turns to me, a slight misting on her face. "Didn't bring an umbrella, did you?"

The water streams down my face, but I keep my eyes on her and say nothing.

"*Purge me with hyssop, and I shall be clean,*" she says, finally.

"What the hell's hyssop?"

She holds the hood around her face and walks faster. When we get to the heavy glass doors of Nordstrom, she stops. I see the two of us mirrored back, her hooded and dry, me uncovered, straggly haired, and soaked.

"Beats me," Jo says. "But my advice for aging DGs is this: dial up your Deadlies. I'd go for #2, Gluttony. Lowest I'd go would be Sloth, #4. But you won't listen; you'll stick with the worst, the bottom circle, the closest to hell." She pushes us into the heavenly pollen-free air of Nordstrom. "Pride, #7. Endemic to doctors of all persuasions. Necessary, maybe. Found in do-gooders too. Doctor do-gooders are the worst."

We stand, dripping on the marble floor. I'm not sure I agree with Jo, but I could go for Gluttony. I eye the golden display of Godivas. Jo heads for the shoes. I think I can smell the dark, rich scent of chocolate—caramels, ganaches, truffles, pralines—right through my stuffed-up nose. The salivary glands begin to do their thing.

No, no, no, I think, turning away. Stereotypes. I cannot ignore that Elephant in the Living Room. I sigh. Jo is the serene goddess, but I'm going to hell in a handbasket.

I turn back and walk over to a large box of truffles. I run my finger across the embossed top. I feel the calories slither toward me. As long, I think, as you're headed to the bottom basement, what's a lingering visit or two along the way? I slide my hands around the box. I carry it to the smiling clerk who waits by the counter.

Lust, Gluttony, Greed, Sloth, Wrath, Envy, Pride. I take a deep breath, pop a chocolate in my mouth, and wave to Jo, who's holding a red stiletto. I've had my epiphany. I hop on the down escalator. Sloth, here I come. Might as well have fun before we turn into screamer-gomeres from the attic, imprisoned in that box they push around the stage. Penitential psalms or not, the play will go on. And we will, all of us—Hippocrates notwithstanding—have caused harm.

May I, I hope, have caused some good, too. Yes, the beginning of Psalm 51: *Have mercy upon us, O God, according to thy loving kindness. . . .*

Maybe the healing we've caused has outweighed the damage.

And in the hidden part thou shalt make me to know wisdom.

Maybe we're old enough, finally.

Wash me thoroughly from mine inequity. O Great God of the House of Men: *make me to hear joy and gladness that the bones which thou hast broken may rejoice.*

Now: on to the next act already.

Rereadings

Chasing Fire Engines

CORTNEY DAVIS

Sometimes, when a soldier Briony was looking after was in great pain, she was touched by an impersonal tenderness that detached her from the suffering, so that she was able to do her work efficiently and without horror. That was when she saw what nursing might be, and she longed to qualify, to have that badge.

IAN MCEWAN, *ATONEMENT*

The secret is to decathect. Withdraw your libidinal investment in what you're doing. It's like putting on a space helmet so that you're not really there. Survival, eh?

SAMUEL SHEM, *THE HOUSE OF GOD*

"OHNOYADONTOHNOYADONTOHNO." A woman's voice emanates from the far end of the clinic hallway and arrives, undiminished, to bounce off the walls of the back room where I'm sitting with three ob-gyn residents and two medical students. I look up from my chart, wondering about the voice or, more precisely, about the patient attached to the voice. A nurse practitioner in the clinic, I've just finished seeing who I thought was the last patient of the day. But looking around the room, I notice one more chart lurking in the to-be-seen rack. Certainly the voice and the chart go together. I glance at my colleagues.

One resident eats an orange, digging his fingers in and ripping the skin, spritzing the pungent spray into the air. Two female residents talk marriage plans and flip through *Bride* magazine. The medical students, looking earnest and a bit like newly hatched birds, are bent over, reading. Furiously highlighting, they hold blue, yellow, and green markers clenched in their fists. No one else seems to see the chart or to hear the voice.

"Hey," I say. "Who's that?" I tip my head toward the chart rack. That little self-righteous part of me wonders if the residents heard me say, "*Who's* that?" not "*What's* that?"

"Crazy old lady," says the orange eater. "Here for her Pap." He turns a big smile my way. "And you know you're so good with them. Anyway, we've got chairman rounds." The residents and students gather their things and, without picking up the orange rinds or the books or the various detritus of their stint in the clinic, walk out. I have a momentary visual image of them one by one picking up the chart, reading the words "Nursing home patient here for Pap," and then gently replacing it in the rack. As they flee from the clinic, the strains of "OHNOYADONTOHNOYADONT" accompany them.

Ah ha, I think to myself. *A gomere.*

I understand. I forgive the residents their youth, their desire for real diseases to cure, their fear of the human unknown, which can turn out to be frighteningly all too familiar. I realize they've probably never read *The House of God.* I must remember to loan them my copy.

The residents' laughter rings in the hallway until it mutes into a ribbon of sound. A nurse opens the door, pokes her head in, and points at the chart. "This patient's been waiting forever. The aide with her wants to know if anyone is ever going to see her."

"Yup," I answer, closing my chart. "I'll be right in."

The House of God found its way into my hands for the first time in 1978, shortly after it was published and just when I was six months into my nurse practitioner training. I'd already worked as an RN for several years in the OR and in the ICU, and as the head nurse on an oncology ward. I was young, eager and naive, as eager and naive as Roy Basch, *The House of God*'s fictional intern and main character. When things were going well, he had "the fantasy of being a real doctor, dealing with real disease" (Shem 179). When I picked up the dangerous arrhythmia or competently pushed IV chemo, I had the fantasy of being the perfect nurse. Now I was going to be a nurse practitioner, moving ever closer to the action. Part of me wanted to comfort, to be always effortlessly kind. Another part of me wanted to be cool and detached, the nurse in white who saved patients from real diseases and then walked away from all that into "real" life.

I thought *The House of God* was the funniest book I'd ever read. When I worked in surgery, I'd identified with the movie *MASH,* and I now identified with the cultlike camaraderie of the men and women of *The House of God.* I felt as if both the movie and this book were written in code, relating an existence only the initiated could understand. In the movie theater watching *MASH* and eating popcorn, my OR colleagues and I had laughed when no one else did—only we insiders got the jokes! When I read about Roy and the Fat Man and Molly and the gomers and gomeres, I felt the same sense of belonging. I was part of a great exclusive club, the magical world of medicine! I knew what it was like, the disappointments and the heroic saves that made it all worthwhile and the strange impersonal eroticism that oozed, at that time, through the hospital halls. Those of us in the know started tossing around words like "buff" and "turf"; we joked with each other about our RORs, relationships on the rocks; we turned a blind eye to the number of residents and physicians having affairs—sometimes a quick peek and squeeze in the linen closet and other times home-wrecking messes. Yes, patients were suffering and, whether we admitted it or not, so were we. Many of us were skating on the surface of our relationships with those in our keeping, never sure how to, or even if we wanted to, dive below the surface.

Reading *The House of God* made the decade's lurking sense of uneasiness seem somehow okay. We really *did* care for our patients, and we really *did* want the best for them, didn't we? All we had to do was remember what the Fat Man said—they were the patients, the ones with the diseases. We were the healthy ones joking in the back room about how the patients' gruesome, suppurating wounds were ruining our appetites and about how the end of a patient's life meant more work for us at the beginning of a shift. This laughter kept us sane—and when we were sane, wasn't there something *fun* about all this, and didn't we, in the end, do a better job?

We knew what Roy and Chuck and the Runt knew—that we'd better put on that House of God space helmet to protect ourselves from getting too close to our patients. Darn them, they always died or else got better and went home, either way leaving us behind. Too often, we didn't know what to do for them and couldn't save them. Or we saved the ones who should have died and made mistakes with the ones who should have lived. Didn't this book prove that we belonged to a rarified group of souls who must be beaten and battered into shape, even if the shape was one we didn't particularly like?

Looking back, I was, for the most part, the kind, efficient nurse I meant to be. I survived numerous astounding moments with patients, life-and-death moments in surgery, in the ICU, and on the oncology ward, moments that, if I let them creep into my consciousness, might wrench the ground from under my feet and set my heart to pounding, my body to trembling. It never occurred to me that I was beginning to turn into two people: the good, efficient nurse who excelled at her work and the very stressed woman who wasn't doing so well in her private life. I missed the whole point of the book. I was young. I was eager. I never read beyond chapter 17.

This is a memory. Picture, if you will, a particular patient on a particular day. She is a young woman, a "frequent flyer" on our oncology ward, someone who's had leukemia for five years but recently seems to be in remission. Then this day she comes into the hospital and, unexpectedly, dies. I am the head nurse.

By then, I'd seen a lot of patients die. I don't mean I'd seen a lot of dead patients, although that's true too. I mean that I'd been with many patients at the precise moment of their death. Death can be a long process, taking months. It can be a short process, taking only a few hours. But always there is that very second in which human life ceases. It is a terrifying privilege to be with someone at the time of this passing.

I am with this young woman when she dies. Her whole dying—if you don't count the years of chemotherapy, relapse, and remission—takes thirty minutes.

I crank up her bed, slide the oxygen prongs into her nostrils. She has lapsed into unconsciousness, and beads of perspiration gather on her forehead as she works to die. Her jaw is slack and falls open, like a puppet's, with each deep guttural breath, more a series of moanings. Soon her doctor comes in, and a respiratory therapist. We all know this patient well; if we allow ourselves a certain uncomfortable familiarity, we might call her our friend. She has dark short hair and smooth skin, freckles over the bridge of her nose. Some people become beautiful in their dying, but she is not one of these. Her family is out of town.

After she dies, the doctor goes out to the nurse's desk to write in her chart. The respiratory therapist shuts off the oxygen and throws away the used tubing.

I am overwhelmed by her dying. My throat burns; I feel dizzy, vertiginous. I think I might vomit or faint. I busy myself with the details death leaves in its aftermath. What will happen if I take off the space helmet of distance and detachment? What if I dare feel not simply an impersonal tenderness but a true tenderness, one that allows me to admit that my patients and I are separated only by the thin line of health, and that their stories are really only the shadow side of my own—that during the hours or days of our acquaintance I don't just care *for* them, I care *about* them? It takes every ounce of my effort, of my strength, not to cry.

Day by day, month by month, the tension between my nursing experiences and my inability *to connect* with those experiences begins to feel like Roy Basch's ROR fight with his girlfriend, Berry: "Our fight was not the violent, howling, barking fight that keeps alive vestiges of love, but that tired, distant, silent fight where fighters are afraid to punch for fear the punch will kill" (141).

There are so many patients hiding at the back of my mind. I do so want to bear witness both to their suffering and to my own. At the same time, I wonder if that witnessing will be the punch that kills me.

Sometimes single events—no matter how many of them and no matter how dramatic—don't have the power to change your life. More often lives change when one event, one happening, triggers the memory of another, perhaps more distant occurrence. Then the two come clashing together, like cymbals, and startle you into a third and new understanding. These two events might be separated by years, by decades.

Recently, I reread *The House of God*. I didn't find it funny anymore. That heady, ironic look at patients that once seemed so pertinent was no longer a part of my reality. The sexual prowess and adventures of the oversexed and overworked interns seemed repetitious, ultimately deadening. I found the treatment of nurses as "recess," as in-house diversion, disturbing. The suffering of the patients, the suffering of the interns, was profoundly unsettling. At last, my eyes were opened to the deeper story behind the story. At last, I read beyond chapter 17.

Somewhere near the end of chapter 22 I found this: "To repair, to re-create the human took some time" (329). And in chapter 26, almost at the book's end, I read how Roy's lover, Berry, sums up Roy's first year in the House of God: "This might have been the only thing that could have awakened you. Your whole life has been a growing from the outside, mastering the challenges that others have set for you. Now, finally, you might just be growing from the inside yourself. It can be a whole new world, Roy, I know it. A whole new life" (379).

Roy changed during his year at the House of God. Something happened to change me too when, years after her death, I wrote a poem about my leukemia patient who died when we least expected it. The poem wasn't triggered by her death. I don't remember precisely when the impulse to write about her came to me, but I know it was initiated by something I saw in the hospital, perhaps an elderly patient alone in a room, her hand raised in the air as if she were reaching for someone. Suddenly all the deaths, all the sufferings, all the humiliations of illness, all the helplessness and dread during the years when I was first learning came back to me and then came together in my remembered images of my patient's death. For so many years of my own internship in the larger house of medicine, I'd thought, like the young doctors in the House of God, that there might somewhere be a magic formula that would both cure my patients and keep me safe; that words like "gomer" and "gomere" could lighten the load and somehow keep me both functioning and untouched. The only container for all this emotion, for me, turned out to be the shape of a poem; for Samuel Shem, it was the shape of a book.

It wasn't my patient's death or the writing of the poem but the two in combination that led me into new territory. All the fears I had about truly being present to a patient's story—and therefore facing my own story as a caregiver—were transformed by the writing of that poem. I think something similar must have happened to Samuel Shem when he wrote *The House of God* and then emerged from behind his pen name to be revealed as Steve Bergman. Surely he had written what he himself experienced in internship; surely he had written his way out of hiding, moving from curing to caring and at last to revelation.

Bergman says he now understands things about *The House of God* that he didn't when he first wrote it. Once after a lecture a student asked, "How could you write this and survive?" In a new afterword to *The House of God,* Bergman says, "I'm not sure how I answered, then. Now I would say, 'Writing this is a way to survive, and to heal'" (397).

My patient is nearing ninety—housebound, gray hair like a crown of spun glass, ankles as thin as a deer's, living in a small four-room house that belongs to her son, who has moved very far away. Visiting her, opening her always-unlocked door, I am always caught by surprise by the deep scent of antique furniture and the passage of time. There is the world outside: bright sun and crisp air, my Subaru parked at her curb. There is her world: the luncheon sandwich and cold dinner dropped off by Meals on Wheels, the old-fashioned silk stockings she pulls on every day and fastens to her garter belt, the two round crescents of rouge she rubs on her cheeks the Thursdays I come to check her, the bed made by her two-hour-a-day aide, the quiet tick of her alarm clock, the pile of magazines and the box of tissues at her bedside. She is as frail as a humming-bird. I love her.

Her hearing is excellent. Before I am all the way inside, she calls out, "Oh, you're here! You're here!" Never have I been greeted with such unabashed de-light. I carry my medical bag through the living room into her small bedroom. Propped up in bed in a sweater set and pleated skirt, a strand of pearls at her throat and a cameo brooch on her lapel, she is a lady smelling of a light perfume, one I never do get the name of. She is alert and alive and so glad to see me. One day, God willing, I will be like her.

I never do much at all to help her. In this the Fat Man had it right—the less I do, the better she will be. Her blood pressure is remarkably stable; her heart sounds are distant but regular; her lungs are clear. She has no edema, a fairly good appetite considering she gets no exercise, and she maintains a lively interest in the world events she watches on TV. I suspect her nights must be very long. Sitting with her, talking with her, making her laugh, watching her become flushed and coy again, I feel my heart opening. Perhaps someday I will write about her, even if that writing might strike others as mundane: an old lady, eventually to die; an old woman who will soon be found cold in her bed. If I write about her, I will find a way to survive her loss. If I write about her story, about any patient's story, I will better live within my own. I know that Steve Bergman discovered this in the writing of *The House of God*—it is the fearless, honest mingling of our stories, caregivers and patients, that leads us beyond curing to vulnerability and then to caring, to healing.

As we sit talking, my patient and I are interrupted by the sudden undulating wail of a siren. She raises her hand to shush me. She leans forward in her bed.

She tells me how, when she was a child, she and her father would run from their house to chase the fire engines. Her eyes glitter. It is a moment of grace. "Oh," she says. "Let's see where it's going! Let's you and I go after it!"

WORKS CITED

McEwan, Ian. *Atonement*. New York: Anchor Books, 2003.
Shem, Samuel. *The House of God*. New York: Delta Trade, 2003.

Speaking the Unspeakable

JAY BARUCH

I put off reading *The House of God* until my fourth year of medical school. Even without cracking the cover I still knew about gomers, the laws of the House of God, the Rose Room, the art of buffing and turfing, the O and Q signs. They were the lingua franca of the medical wards. An occasional student would carry the book around, wearing a devious, knowing grin, as if it were forbidden fruit or a magical drug. Even if the book punctured the idealized world sold to us by medical school professors, I made a conscious decision not to read it, wary of what I might discover inside and what it might do to me.

As it is with most fun things that carry risk or the allure of corruption, I could resist *The House of God* for only so long. I dove into the experience. Reading became a violently physical act. I laughed. I squirmed. I self-righteously shook my head. But I also found the term "gomer" offensive and insensitive, the laws too clever. I didn't identify with any of the interns, which made it much easier to convince myself that what happened to them wouldn't happen to me. The sharp, energized prose and vividly outrageous scenes left me breathless with admiration. But in the end I was disappointed with the book, which was a great relief.

That changed when my emergency medicine residency began. I could no longer pretend the emotions, judgments, and behaviors that I had criticized in the book weren't embedded in me.

New words crept easily into my vocabulary. The demented, moaning Jewish woman was in Oy-tach. The overly theatrical Hispanic woman was in Status Hispanicus. The homeless, chronically inebriated frequent flyer brought into the ER during bitterly cold winters was a Drunksicle. We referred to the unresponsive gomer as gomertose. We'd shake our heads, chuckle furtively. I recognized such objectifying language as insensitive and denigrating. But at the same time, this vocabulary from tired, insecure, frightened physicians-in-training felt necessary and strangely comforting.

I soon discovered there weren't enough rationalizations and pints of beer in the world to help make sense of how, again and again, *I* disappointed *myself.*

Forget the sanitized and deeply moral approach to doctor-patient relationships taught in medical schools, with a focus on neutered patient personalities that serve you well if you're in a classroom, well rested and dealing with intellectual constructions. Some patients evoke uncomfortable feelings in their caregivers—suspicion, doubt, distrust, even dislike. Some yell, smell, or test the limits of the kindest staff. They blame us and we blame them. The 500-pound diabetic with abdominal pain. The two-pack-a-day smoker who comes to the hospital gasping for air on a regular basis. The drunks who fall down, sober up, and get sent home only to come back a few hours later with enough alcohol in their blood to kill most people. Sometimes patients are simply too needy. These patients are the toughest, looking to me for answers when I don't have any.

Such thoughts make me uncomfortable. Confessing them openly feels criminal, unsavory. But it's important to be transparent and blunt. *The House of God* is filled with moments and insights that are so honest they feel obscene. Listen to Dr. Roy Basch on his emergency ward rotation:

> I got competent to handle the big stuff, and the other stuff is just one abusive person after another. It shits. Addicts trying to dupe you for dope, drunks, the poor, the clap, the lonelies—I hate 'em all. I don't trust anyone. It comes from being vomited on and spit at and yelled at and conned. Everyone's out to get me to do something for them, for their fake disease. The first thing I look for now is how they're trying to take me for a ride. It's paranoia, see? (208)

What emergency physician or nurse hasn't entertained such thoughts from time to time? These raw, politically incorrect feelings are difficult for one to acknowledge or discuss without being perceived by others as someone who is unprofessional, burnt out, or short on the commitment or toughness required to work in the Emergency Department.

Critics have accused the book of being racist, misogynistic, and ageist, among other things. There may be passages where these charges have some grounding, but not the work as a whole. If it's judgmental in any way, it's only because doctors and health care providers can't avoid passing judgment, having opinions and prejudices. What's important isn't ridding them of their personal views, but ensuring that doctors and doctors-in-training have the insight and sensitivity to recognize and reflect upon them, and enough equipoise and emotional commitment that it doesn't interfere with patient care.

I loved the scene when Dr. Roy Basch watches the Fat Man shovel day-old blintzes into his mouth while the two of them are on call. The Fat Man is talking, and Roy can't be sure he isn't listening to a ranting madman. "I'm not crazy," Fats says, "it's just that I spell out what every other doc feels, but most squash down and let eat away at their guts. Last year I lost weight. Me! So I said to myself, 'Not your gastric mucosa, Fats baby, not for what they're paying you. No ulcer for you'" (76).

As a medical student, I was taught to learn from my mistakes, but it was infinitely better to learn from the mistakes of others. When I first read *The House of God,* I didn't know what to make of the Fat Man. My opinion fluctuated from awe and amazement to deep-seated concern. He seemed too hip, too distracted—an operator. But the second time around I snapped to attention whenever he appeared on the page. He has a sharp, cutting eye on the many storms the young doctors faced and knows how to negotiate them to preserve his sanity and his life. Roy Basch is fortunate to have Fats, who has not only practical wisdom and insight but the interest and desire to share it. And what to make of all his sarcasm? "So who isn't sarcastic? Docs are no different from anyone else, they just pretend they're different?" (192).

And time hasn't dulled the bite in his sarcasm. One can argue that some of the Fat Man's exhortations—for example, that sometimes it's better to do nothing, and "the cure is the disease" (193)—are ominously prescient thirty years later, with widespread antibiotic resistance to common bacteria; the emergence of methicillin-resistant staphylococcus, a once hospital-based infection, in the community; and the U.S. Institute of Medicine report that illuminated the shocking number of deaths that occur each year in hospitals due to medical error.

The veracity of the Fat Man's perceptions isn't what I admire most about him now. It's his ferocious honesty. His balance, his integrity, his authenticity. His courage to break ranks with the establishment. Roy Basch tells him at the end, "But you showed me that a guy can still stay in medicine and still be himself" (338).

You can't become a doctor or a nurse and think that all the sharp edges in your personality, the trapdoors and dead ends that complicate your opinions of others, will suddenly vanish or smooth out. If anything, the stresses of being intimate with people and their lives and problems will only test the strength and validity of your beliefs.

I remember frantically treating a patient, Mr. X, who was barely breathing. His skin was gray, moving toward blue. We couldn't get an IV in his scarred veins; there were surgical scars on his neck. Intubation, placing a breathing tube in his trachea, must have been as difficult in the past as it was now. He had pinpoint pupils. We assumed he was a narcotic overdose. But the intramuscular nalaxone wasn't working. A second-year medical student was shadowing me for the day, and I could feel the force of his gaze as everything I did failed, and confidence bled from the room. The nurses and I spoke in tense, sober glances.

I ordered a last dose of nalaxone. Anesthesia was on the way. I set up for a cricothyroidotomy. I tried to hide the white fear, the cool trembling in my bones.

Mr. X might die. The nurses were two of my favorites. Caring, funny, clinically outstanding. They were all business now, their tone fraying with panic.

Then Mr. X bolted upright on the stretcher, coughing, red eyes bulging. The nalaxone had finally kicked in. He scratched himself, shivered. The hairs on his arms stood at attention. All signs of narcotic withdrawal, which is what we precipitated by giving the reversal drug. He denied overdosing. He denied using heroin or any other narcotics. He scoffed, appeared offended by our questions.

A grateful sigh swept through the room like a cool, easy breeze. Then one of the nurses mumbled under her breath disgustedly, "I know him."

"Oh," said the other nurse, recognizing Mr. X.

The mood took a dark turn. Mr. X had overdosed on heroin several times in the past few months. I now recognized him, too.

"He overdosed once in front of his kids," someone said. "He's real trash."

"Trash?" I thought to myself, cringing.

We were standing at the nursing station now, shaking our heads, a fair distance away from the patient. I feared for the example we were setting for the medical student, who had been with us, listening to every word. Did we seem regretful that our diligent work had saved this particular man, or that we cared so intensely for a man whom we later learned couldn't care less about himself or his family? Did we give the impression that saving this man's life was a bad outcome?

We shared our private thoughts in an impromptu and surprisingly candid dialogue, shattering all pretense of sensitivity expected of health care providers. The nurses knew Mr. X's wife and other family members. They shared stories too harsh and heartbreaking to be true. When the conversation was over, I felt closer to my colleagues. We weren't any more accepting of Mr. X, but we achieved enough workable resignation to allow ourselves to shrug our shoulders, take a deep breath, and reclaim our compassion.

Mr. X began barking, demanding to go home. The nurses screwed on smiles and dutifully attended to him. I spoke with the medical student about what he had witnessed, treating Mr. X and the conversation that followed. Then we walked over to speak with Mr. X, who didn't want to talk with me. He didn't care that we had saved his life. If anything, he seemed pissed about that. I let him scream and yell. The nalaxone would soon wear off. Ideally, he'd soon drop off to sleep and still breathe comfortably.

The great challenge educating physicians-in-training is balancing hope, optimism, and encouragement with an appropriate dose of realism and honesty to adequately prepare them for the demands of patient care in the current health care environment.

Medical school and residencies are often approached as time-limited experiences to be endured, but many of these issues follow young physicians far into their careers. The doctor-patient interaction can be beautiful, fragile, and unsteady, a source of comfort, frustration, or fireworks.

When Dr. Sanders is dying, he says to Dr. Roy Basch, "What sustains us is when we find a way to be compassionate, to love" (156). Later, Roy recognizes that "I knew that I could not do what Dr. Sanders had told me to do, to 'be with' others. I could not 'be with' others, for I was somewhere else, in some cold place, insomniac in the midst of dreamers, far far from the land of love" (287).

Doctoring places great demands on the brain but asks more from the heart. It's an emotional contact sport. Medical students, residents, practicing physicians, and other health care providers should never feel "somewhere else." A vital part of medical education must be devoted to nurturing reflective skills and shaping the space so they can share feelings and experiences that often are passed over in doctoring. Medical educators must learn to "be with" students and residents in a way that is pragmatic and honest. A reversal agent has yet to be invented to treat the "insomniac." Until then, we're left with *The House of God,* and all its breadth, wisdom, and heresy to help guide us. It might offend some people, maybe even be considered obscene by teachers and students alike, but it's offensive and obscene because, like medicine, it's filled with humanity.

NOTES

Citations in the text refer to the Delta Trade Paperback, 2003 edition.

Shem Redux: Is It time?

STEVEN HYMAN

My return to Samuel Shem's *The House of God* after a period of many years elicited potent memories of my medical internship and of the general hospital of the late twentieth century. The vivid descriptions of the experiences of medical intern Roy Basch and his colleagues at a Boston teaching hospital in the mid-1970s remain emotionally evocative today. Shem portrays a series of disturbing episodes across the calendar year of internship, including an intern's suicide, and conveys the interminable grind of an intern's life. As *The House of God* takes one through various inpatient wards, the emergency ward, and the intensive care unit, there is a devastating cumulative effect. The growing fatigue, the growing distance between the interns and their outside lives, the growing dehumanization of patients all take a severe toll. From some perspectives the internship portrayed by Shem can seem like its own chronic illness. For those of us who lived through similar "schooling," the book has the power to bring back not only cognitive recollections but also visceral experiences that have been stored away somewhere in our brains: feelings of intense fatigue or of the emotional disinhibition produced by sleeplessness, foul smells, and close contact with agony and death.

On the surface this is a sardonic exposé, complete with Joycean commentators in the persons of the clever policemen, Gilheeny and Quick, lest we miss any dark detail. At its heart, however, *The House of God* is a bildungsroman in which Basch passes through a kind of hell to reach a new level of understanding and maturity, albeit not without lasting scars. The theme of a passage through hell necessarily contributes to the selection of stories told. These are stories of the dehumanization of elderly demented patients, of the intern Potts being driven to suicide, of the need for Basch to drive over the stains left by Potts's fallen body to park at the hospital every day, of the mercenary motivations of some of the private physicians. While a selection, not the totality, of the internship, these stories are not wild fantasies, and the experiences of internship would provide much grist for Shem's trip through hell.

For Shem's approximate contemporaries, of whom I am one, the 1970s setting, with the Watergate hearings as a riveting foil to all else, brought with it a heightened distrust of authority. In medicine, as in all professions, this distrust was partly warranted. It was a time when authority asserted on the basis of status was no longer accepted without question and in which young people wanted to know why the world worked a certain way. *The House of God* punctures the defenses of many a tradition and many an authority figure that warranted such treatment. That said, the book seems almost relentlessly dark. For all the humorless, narcissistic martinets that populated my internship, there were also smart, erudite, yet still empathic doctors to learn from. Put another way, I had more than the Fat Man and my wife to lean on and learn from. That said, against the background of exhaustion and stress, the bad guys really did tend to stand out. Much of the conversation among the interns and residents of my day, in my Boston teaching hospital, was survival talk. Not surprisingly, tales of abuse and horror, of the venality and dangerousness of some of the "society docs," could be heard any night at the late dinner served to those on call. Dark humor became a kind of salvation, because it could hold naked anger or depression at bay. The experience of working so hard in mortal situations, with so little experience and so little rest, did not always bring out the best in us. Sardonic laughter was a very effective defense, so long as it did not turn to cynicism or grease the slippery slope toward the dehumanization of patients. Some people argue over who should populate the all-time all-star baseball team. We argued over who among the society docs could rightfully be considered for a place among the four horsemen of the apocalypse. If consensus were reached on that matter, we would go on to spirited disagreements over the next tier, the pretenders to a place among the horsemen, whom we called the ponies of the apocalypse. An outsider hearing us would have thought we had gone mad. In fact, we were just trying to manage a surfeit of emotion so that we could finish our greasy, calorie-laden dinner and go on.

It is remarkable how universal the kinds of experiences described in *The House of God* are. Even though I was not a medical intern at the House, but at the equally thinly disguised MBH, some episodes were eerily similar. For example, in *The House of God*, a surgical resident prays for the arrival of extremely ill and challenging patients as a way of proving his mettle. As I read this episode, I was transported to the rear of the emergency ward during my internship, where my bright, aggressive, and success-oriented medical resident looked up to the heavens one night, extended his arms with his palms turned up in supplication, and prayed for the deity to send us the sickest possible train wreck so that we could "show our stuff." I thought this was insane because the alternative was to get a few hours' sleep. My recollection is that he got his wish and, as a result, sleep evaded us. I remember feeling that this very bright resident brought a paramilitary demeanor to the practice of hospital medicine. He was punctilious on rounds, able to rattle off eponyms like a machine gun, and hungry for opportunities to perform invasive procedures. Sadly for him, our hospital did not value starched white coats; he would have loved them. Certainly, both he and I were too aggressive at times in our interventions. As in the House, no one was going to die with abnormal chemistries if we could help it. Undoubtedly, the quest for perfection sometimes warped our judgment. My resident's marinelike assault on the beachhead of disease notwithstanding, his medical judgment was generally excellent, and he was unfailingly polite, almost preternaturally so with patients. We all had our defense mechanisms in the strange, stressful, frightening, sleepless world of the hospital. The key was to attack the disease, but not the poor soul who had it. *The House of God* makes clear that it may be easy to say that is the key. It is very hard to think and act that way under the circumstances, and without the support of mentors and loved ones, it is very easy to lose one's way.

In *The House of God*, Basch emerges from his year wiser and ready to move on after taking a year to recuperate, but the clear implication is that not everyone achieves wisdom. The question lurking in my mind as I read was whether American medicine as a whole has become wiser and more humane over the last three decades. The evidence is mixed, but the trouble is not entirely intrinsic to medicine. I do not mean that doctors, clinics, hospitals, and all the components of the health care system should be let off the hook. I only mean that different components of American society are engaged in a confused dance with the medical system. We want only the best for our loved ones, while we demand that medicine reduce its costs. We want humane care for the dying, but we also want to preserve life at all costs. We want to relieve the terrible pain of cancer, but we worry (insanely) about fostering addictions among the dying and (less insanely) about the misuse of narcotics by drug abusers posing as patients.

With steady progress in technology, we have a far greater ability to keep hearts beating at all costs than when *The House of God* was written. On the positive side of the ledger there is a healthy and growing movement to encourage people to write advance directives so that when the time comes to die, they might be permitted to do so. Although a hospice provokes distress in Basch at the end of the book, it is good to have alternatives to aggressive treatment at the end of life, an alternative to what we as interns called "flogging" the dying patient.

The cost cutting that has decreased the number of hospital beds means that the wards can no longer serve as an ersatz sandbar for marooned elderly and disabled patients. That does not mean, however, that their care is more humane. It also means that the numbers of admissions and discharges faced by today's Roy Basches are of dizzying proportions. I suspect that much would be different were Roy Basch to begin his internship again, some of it clearly better, but much of it not. Maybe Samuel Shem needs to take a sabbatical from what he is doing and spend a bit of time chronicling what is happening on the wards today.

The House of God *Redux*

THOMAS DUFFY

Samuel Shem's eschatological novel, *The House of God*, has achieved classic status for its merciless and often hilarious description of house staff training in an academic medical center in the 1970s. It challenged with unabashed ribaldry and Animal House–like humor the often inhuman demands of residency training at that time. The ignoble aspects of a noble profession were exaggerated, but the novel strongly resonated with the lived experiences of many physicians of that period. The young physicians' scorn for any perceived cant or lack of authenticity, their fluency in a rich language of colorful terms used to characterize patients and parody teachers, and the sexual frenzy of the fleeting couplings between doctors and nurses all contributed to an irreverent but honest portrayal of this rite of passage in a "sacred" profession. Sick humor sustained these wounded healers, but not without significant coarsening of their moral sensibilities and an emotional removal from their patients. Just as in many other medical training programs, some careers and even lives were prematurely ended by the pressures of the bonding and bondage that internship appeared to encourage.

The House of God became required reading, almost a cult literature for members of the profession and medical students. Its colorful assortment of acronyms was adopted as part of the medical vernacular, a means of categorizing and highlighting the worst features of particular patient populations and diseases. The word "gomer," an acronym for "Get out of my emergency room," became the patois in many hospitals; the acronym conveyed how perverted the doctor-patient relationship had become for these young physicians. Moral leadership was absent in the House of God, where the chief of medicine was an object of the most cruel caricature for his insensitivity to his charges' sufferings. It was a place where Roy, the main character, euthanizes a patient, an act that is depicted as driven by misplaced compassion originating in a physician's frustration and exhaustion. The "hidden" curriculum, the unacknowledged tribal behavior of the beleaguered house officers, bore no relationship or resemblance to the idealized curriculum described in old-fashioned novels by Sinclair Lewis or A. J. Cronin. The unrelenting encounters with concentrated tragedy quenched any lifeblood of idealism and virtue the young physicians had brought with them to doctoring; the euphemistic House of God had become a hell house.

My initial readings of the novel ended prematurely on several occasions, before I had completed the book; I felt sullied and soiled by the events and behavior depicted therein. I had brought to the book my own house staff training experience in a different institution from a decade earlier. The workload and the hours required in my training superseded even those of Shem's era, but expectations that physicians be gentlemen (there were few women) still remained in effect and on display. Our chief embodied this ideal, and his example and quiet but firm command guaranteed this way of life for all of us. There were episodes of grossness at patients' expense that arose out of the circumstances of young physicians' lives. One evening an intern broadcast a loud belch through the public address system of the patients' rooms. When confronted regarding this silly gaffe and threatened with discipline, he began to weep. The situation was different from its initial interpretation as a prank inserting bathroom humor into the medical setting. His comedic bellowing was not a flatulent joke, but rather a cry of anguish, a peal of frustration with the circumstances of his life as an intern. This kind of misbehavior was not common. My co-interns were remarkably compliant with the iron-man expectations of our leaders, and we internalized these traits for ourselves. We chose to remain in internal medicine. Those who opted out were perceived as not possessing the "right stuff." We persevered in the medical residency and imposed the same performance standards on our successors. We were not yet aware that a lasting impact and debt were being incurred by our failure to acknowledge and deal with the cost of training in a medical environment that was unlike the House of God but still shared with it a form of training that plunged young physicians into waters far above their heads.

A recent return to the book in its new edition changed my reaction and reading of the book. The text was the same, but I, the physician-reader, brought a changed person to the encounter. Although the distance in time was lengthy and I felt far removed from that period in my life, certain events and aspects of house staff training were more vivid and more comprehensible to me. The novel heightened those memories, many of which were traumatic and still imprinted on me. I had not forgotten the bungled lumbar puncture that cost a patient's life, the mix-up of potassium chloride for saline that resulted in a cardiac arrest, the suicide of a woman whose anguish I had overlooked, perhaps because I was too overwhelmed by my own unvisited anguish. Back then, I berated myself for many weeks for my failure to recognize early eclampsia as the cause of a young woman's headaches; her arrival near the end of my twenty-four-hour shift was not an acceptable excuse for my diagnostic error. My experiences, devoid of the

Animal House antics of the novel, still shared with Shem's the same unrelenting encounters with horrors, the same sleep-deprived periods, and the same soil for maladjustments in the future.

The House of God concludes with the end of the internship year. Most of the intern group has chosen to seek some surcease in psychiatry training. They are removing themselves from harm's way by choosing away from a life in internal medicine. Roy has placed even greater distance between himself and the House of God; he has traveled to France, he has bid adieu to a world that has caused him to lose his idealism for medicine and to become bitter over the circumstances that caused that loss. His black bag, his badge as a physician, becomes a discus that he fiercely launches as a symbol of his release from the House of God and all it represents. The launch does not rid him of the torments that remain festering, even in the midst of his European idyll. The events of his internship have been incorporated into his emotional DNA, and no splicing will offer a simple or rapid expulsion of the baggage he now carries. Shem's description of his character's flashbacks and violent nightmares depicts a man suffering with post-traumatic stress in the aftermath of medicine as warfare. His co-interns' subsequent journeys are not detailed. Their year has ended but its aftermath may have created a purgatory in its wake.

That purgatory is soon experienced by Roy even though he has voyaged to the vineyards and beaches of France in the sweet embrace of his loving partner and confidant, Berry. The events and traumas of his residency year continue to invade and discolor the landscape of his new idyll. Gomers now keep company with succulent artichokes; the fine finger control necessary for deflowering the tasty, downy center are beyond the dexterity of aged French gomers. Erotic daydreams lose their heatedness as thoughts of Cooper's ligament intrude on the voluptuousness of bouncing breasts. Sexual couplings become frantic fantasias of fornication amidst the bloody carnage of an unsuccessful cardiac resuscitation. Booze becomes Roy's anodyne to blot out the flashbacks, the intrusive thoughts, the anxiety, and the hyperexcitability that remain the residue of his baptism in the fires of internship. All the features were in place for Roy's purgatory to progress to a hellish life, a fate that has befallen other physicians in similar circumstances. A bad seed has been planted that might crowd out the roots and durability needed to sustain a life in medicine.

There is no shortage of descriptions of physicians whose lives have unraveled in the midst of ministering to others. Alcoholism, drug addiction, and suicide are occupational hazards in the medical profession; the relative risks for suicide are as high as 3.4 in male physicians and 5.7 in female physicians. The major risk factors for suicide are mental disorders and substance abuse. Personal and professional losses, financial problems, a tendency to overwork, and career dissatisfaction are additional factors thought contributory to suicide. Explanations have been sought in the identification of flaws in the individuals who never realized their potential, or of any shortcomings, vulnerabilities, excessive sensitivity, and any weakness of character that may have contributed to lost or mangled lives. Very little consideration has been given to extrinsic factors that might play an even more significant role in creating the shadows that give way to darkness in physicians' lives. My rereading of *The House of God* discovers a narrative of those causal factors; the real power and prescience of the novel are in its depiction of the unacceptable cost and casualties of some medical training.

Potts's suicide in the House of God leaves his co-interns "stunned, numb, and too scared to cry" (328). Roy places the responsibility for the suicide in the failure of his superiors to recognize Potts's suffering. The institution had cultivated an atmosphere where "denying hope and fear, ritualized defenses pulled up around ears like turtlenecks, these doctors, to survive had become machines, sealed off from humans . . . from the warmth of compassion and the thrill of love . . . this internship—this whole training—it destroys people" (328). Others, like Chuck, carry a bottle of Jack Daniels in their black bags as a means to obliterate or soften the harsh realities of their encounters. Roy continues to use alcohol as an escape that could become an addiction, as it has for many other physicians in similar circumstances. The Fat Man possesses greater resiliency amidst the carnage, but he has traded a cynic's role for the healer's role. The closing chapters of the book contain no fairy-tale ending; the characters do not necessarily live happily thereafter. The wounds inflicted by this form of training can continue to fester and drain the wounded healer of his idealism in medicine.

The House of God was published in 1978; it was only in the 1980s that stress reactions were first recognized as the post-Vietnam syndrome. Its features had been described in earlier war stories such as *The Red Badge of Courage,* but war is not its only precipitant. More recently it has been documented that the disorder occurs after bone marrow and cardiac transplants; burn victims and their caregivers, medics, and firefighters are all candidates for stress disorders. Hospitals, like MASH units, are settings where one is exposed to events that are outside the range of normal human experience and that would be markedly distressing to almost anyone. In addition to this critical exposure, individuals with stress disorders often manifest a strong emotional reaction such as fear, terror, or hopelessness. This may be difficult to identify in physicians since imperturbability, the fabled equanimitas of medicine, may fool even us into believing that we are not threatened by what it is we encounter. The absence of institutional investment in helping young physicians to recognize this threat and avert its happening still remains; its occurrence at a temporal remove from the period of training may also contribute to its nonrecognition. Alcoholism and drug addiction may masquerade as primary problems, but they are likely the maladaptive habits unwisely used to cope with the refuse of the past.

Shem, in his afterword to his novel, paraphrases Chekhov's observation that the best writers describe life as it should be in addition to life as it is. The novel is characterized by Updike as farce, but it is farce in its powerful role as a gadfly in prodding the reader to address medical training as it should be. The Libby Zion case is cited as a precipitant of the movement that led to the eighty-hour workweek ruling, even though *The House of God* vividly described the toll of sleep deprivation many years earlier. The book also anticipated the concerns of the nascent field of bioethics, which casts a cold eye on the behavior of physicians in their interactions with patients and their colleagues. The corrosive effect of residency training on the moral compass of young physicians has markedly lessened; the hidden curriculum that was part of most hospitals' culture was outed in the book, contributing to a saner and more humane system of training. *The House of God* gave voice to the previously stifled cries of "wooden men in rusty ships" as they sallied forth as young physicians in America (Rogers 212).

Training of physicians has been mollified and chastened; physicians are now less burdened by scars incurred in exhausting training programs. But new currents in medicine may create the substrate for the writing of farces satirizing the next generation of medical training. The acronyms of "turfing" and "gomer" have been conjoined with "groping" (getting rid of patients) as the essential survival techniques of the house officer. There is now a constant effort and pressure to shorten the hospital stays of patients, an undertaking of which hospital administrations have been the most vocal enthusiasts. This pass-through phenomenon may cancel out the gains of the eighty-hour workweek. The volume of critically ill patients in modern hospitals has greatly increased, and the gap between learning and service by house officers has narrowed. Stress has not been eliminated by the new work-hour restrictions; it has simply been redistributed. Although it is unlikely that the excesses of *The House of God* will recur, the novel has left a heritage that should force the profession to care for its students and young physicians with the same care it delivers to its patients. Otherwise there will continue to be casualties in the ranks of wounded healers who choose to adhere to the laws of the House of God.

WORKS CITED

Rogers, D. E. "On Iron Men in Wooden Ships: Some Thoughts on House Staff Training." *Trans Am Clin Climatol Assoc* 96 (1984): 212–16.
Shem, Samuel. *The House of God.* New York: Dell, 2003.

You Gotta Know the Territory:
The House of God *as Job Description*

PERRI KLASS

I want to start with a famous story about the play *Death of a Salesman,* Arthur
Miller's iconic drama of family disconnections and disappointed dreams that
opened on Broadway in 1949. According to this story, at some point during
the initial run, the playwright overheard two real salesmen discussing their
reactions to the tragedy of Willy Loman. One of the salesmen said to the
other: "That New England territory never was any good." Well, or maybe he
said, "I always told you that New England territory wasn't worth a damn."
When I went looking for the original version of this often-told story, I found
multiple published versions, which left me wondering whether this is in fact
an apocryphal story. (I had actually originally been told that the line was "That
New England territory always was a son-of-a-bitch!") But whether it was an
authentic New York theater moment or just a dramaturgical urban legend,
it remains a profound story because of what it says about the occupational
ear: when you hear (or read or watch) a story about your own profession, the
way that you hear (or read or watch) inevitably shifts. There is a professional
perspective that changes the way you tell a story, and it changes the way you
understand a story. To that possibly fictitious salesman, Willy Loman was just
a poor sap stuck with a rotten assignment, a job description that was certain
to grind him down and leave him a loser. Give him a better territory, and his
story would be completely different—and at this point, those of us who draw
our cultural references from the Broadway stage must inevitably imagine the
salesmen in that railway car in the opening scene of *The Music Man* leaning
forward to sing in chorus, "You gotta know the territory!"

So what does this have to do with *The House of God*? Well, to me, *The House
of God* is a book about choosing the right match as a fourth-year medical
student—in other words, a book about why I didn't go into internal medicine.
When I first read it as a medical student, I was hugely relieved. I had done my
first clinical rotation, at the beginning of my third year, in internal medicine
at a tertiary care Harvard teaching hospital. Everyone knew (all the medical
students, that is, and the house staff and the faculty too, I suppose, though
we didn't discuss it with them) that *The House of God* was set on the internal

medicine service of a different Harvard teaching hospital. I had not enjoyed my time in internal medicine, and I was feeling very troubled about how much I had not enjoyed it. All through the first two years of medical school, I had absorbed a medical student ethos of eagerness for clinical exposure. We went to our classes (or didn't go to our classes) and attended our discussion sections and handed in our problem sets—but what we craved, all of us, was what lay beyond. Clinical medicine, the wards, the chance to touch patients and be part of the profession. That was why we were here, that was where we were heading; that was what would make sense of our lives.

And then I didn't like internal medicine, and I wondered whether in fact my life did not make sense. Why was I in medical school, if I didn't like Medicine? Why was I floundering and unhappy in my very first—and probably my most important—clinical rotation? Why did I wake up in the morning feeling a sense of dread, why did I cringe when they sent me to work up a patient, why did I retreat to the bathroom and cry? Had I made a cosmically wrong choice, spent my energy and my effort and my parents' money all to learn that I had battled my way into a world where I didn't want to live?

Now in some ways I know, looking back, that blaming the field of internal medicine for my feelings back in 1984 is like blaming the state of New Jersey for the miseries of being fourteen years old. Being fourteen can be miserable, and I was often miserable when I was fourteen; I was fourteen in New Jersey—does that mean New Jersey was at fault? Well, yes and no, I can't help feeling. I might have been unhappy anywhere, but my own particular miseries were very much suburban New Jersey miseries, and I suspect I won't forgive easily (I mean, I'm about to turn fifty, and I'm still holding a grudge here). So yes, I had lots of reasons for being miserable when I was doing internal medicine as a third-year student: I had just had a baby—he was five months old when I started the rotation—and I was still nursing; therefore, I was chronically sleep deprived and somewhat hormonally unbalanced and very unhappy to find myself working all night every third night. I was doing my very first clinical rotation, and I hadn't taken the trouble to acquire a lot of preparation about what would be expected of me, so I was constantly learning the hard way and feeling like a fool. I was paired with a famously competitive medical student partner who carried various nicknames in our class referring to his killer instincts and, who, it seemed to me, took great delight in humiliating me—not that it was any great challenge to humiliate me. And it was summer, and the interns were new and scared and under lots of pressure, and worried about their own skills, and worried about their patients, and they probably didn't have a lot of time or compassion or energy to spare.

And none of that has anything to do with internal medicine. But even so, when I think about how unhappy I was during those first months on the wards,

I think about how much I didn't belong in internal medicine. And when I first read *The House of God,* I felt vindicated: this is what it's like, I thought. This is why I didn't want to be there. This is why I woke up every morning with a feeling of impending doom.

And you know what? I still reread the book and think, This is why I didn't go into internal medicine. I am still incapable of reading it as a book about the larger truths of life and death, or as a book about the ways that medical training and medical practice can eat away at your soul, or about black humor in the face of death and disease. To me, it is a cautionary tale: think carefully before you match, my children! Beware of tertiary care inpatient adult medicine! That New England territory never was any good.

And the truth is, my own feelings about clinical experiences took a huge and rapid turn for the better as soon as I ventured outside internal medicine. I liked psychiatry—which I had never remotely expected. I loved pediatrics—yes, I felt happy when I woke up in the morning and faced another day on the wards; yes, I was pleased and interested when they told me to go work up another patient. I even liked surgery—by that point in my third year, I had definitely decided to go into pediatrics, but I had a ball during my months of surgery, and I thought that most of what I was doing was totally cool, or, as we say in Boston, wicked awesome. Could you argue that maybe the difference was that I needed to learn a little more about how to be a functional medical student on a clinical rotation, and that once I learned that, I felt more comfortable and more sure of myself and my place in the world, and I got more pats on the back? Could you argue that maybe the difference was that I needed to be a few more months postpartum, a little more certain that my son and I were both doing okay? Could you even argue that maybe the difference was that I had a medical student partner I didn't like, or a resident I didn't get along with on that first rotation, and then went on, by the luck of the draw, to work with people I genuinely liked in other fields? That is all perfectly plausible, but I know what I know: I was doing internal medicine, and I was miserable, QED. And then I went into pediatrics, and I was happy.

So what do I mean? Let me try to identify some of the zones where I felt—where I still feel—that *The House of God* had internal medicine—at least in the Harvard teaching hospitals—perfectly pegged. By and large, they are the same areas where the book feels to me most transgressive and most bold, the moments where I sit back, feeling that something is being said here that had not previously been put into words. I was never particularly shocked by the humor (by the third year of medical school, you're pretty much accustomed to the humor) or by the sex, which I have to admit I assumed was completely fictional (applying the take-what-guys-say-they've-done-and-divide-by-five rule, which we learned, actually, back in New Jersey), or by the various medical locutions, from "LOL in NAD" to "gomer."

But there were elements in the book that did shock me—or that I found shocking. So in the tradition of the laws of the House of God, let me offer five examples of truths disclosed in the book that I found truly transgressive, and truly revelatory in their frankness.

I. "THESE FINGERS DO NOT TOUCH BODIES."

First and foremost, I must admit, was the willing acknowledgment that many aspects of examining patients' bodies, or the products of their bodies, are frankly disgusting. The Fat Man spells it out on his very first appearance in the book.

> "In internal medicine, there is virtually no need to see patients. Almost all patients are better off unseen. See these fingers?"
>
> We looked carefully at the Fat Man's stubby fingers.
>
> "These fingers do not touch bodies unless they have to. You want to see bodies, go see bodies. I've seen enough bodies, and especially bodies of gomers, to last me the rest of my life." (Shem 27–28)

And then, sure enough, when the narrator, Basch, and the other intern, Potts, actually find themselves examining a patient, well. . . .

> "This is the most depressing thing I've ever done," said Potts, lifting up a pendulous breast as Ina continued to shriek and attempt to whack him with her tied-down left hand.
>
> Under the breast was greeny scumlike material, and as the foul aroma hit us, I thought that this first day must be even worse for Potts. (35)

You have to remember how eager most medical students are to learn the physical exam. Even the way we say it, *the* physical exam, suggests the way it is enshrined in the profession—the art of physical diagnosis, the laying on of hands, the privileged and undeniable professional contact that I think most of us mostly believe is at the very core of the doctor-patient relationship. So what do you do with the emotions that the physical exam sometimes conjures up—the reluctance to touch, the sense of repulsion? Among pediatricians, it's a topic we don't often discuss—that many of us went into the field in part because we find it much more pleasant to deal with children's bodies, even when they are sick or hurt. But there is no question in my mind that one reason I was unhappy when they told me to go work up a new internal medicine admission was that

I often did not relish the job of examining another adult body, especially the body of an elderly and severely debilitated patient—I knew the word "gomer," of course, but as a self-consciously humane feminist medical student in the 1980s, I probably wouldn't have used it.

II. "YOU CAN LEARN A LOT FROM THAT AROMA."

And then, a related second truth: medicine stinks. *The House of God* is particularly lyrical on the subject of odor—who can forget the Rose Room, so called because, according to the Fat Man, it inevitably contains four female gomers (the term "gomere" is not one I have encountered elsewhere, but then, of course, I am in pediatrics), all named Rose.

> In hushed silence we stood in the middle of the dimly lit Rose Room. All was still, spectral, the four Roses horizontal, at peace, barely dimpling their swaddling sheets. It was all very nice, until the smell hit, and then it was disgusting. The smell was shit. I couldn't stand it. I left. . . . Finally, out came our leader, asking, "What's the matter, guys?"
>
> We told him the matter was the aroma.
>
> "Yeah, well, you can learn a lot from that aroma. With luck, in three months you'll be able to stand in the middle of that room and give the four diagnoses as the different bowel odors smack your olfactory lobes. Why, just today there was a steatorrheac malabsorption, a bowel carcinoma, a superior mesenteric insufficiency giving rise to bowel ischemia and diarrhea, and last? . . . yes! Little packets of gas slipping past a long-standing fecal impaction." (230–31)

Well, there it is: medicine often stinks. A certain amount of learning to take care of patients involves learning to overcome your sense of revulsion at all the various odors that the human body can produce. No one talks about it in your physical diagnosis class, but smells are part of the job. And speaking of smells, and speaking of revulsion, you have to spend time dealing with all the various unappealing products of the body. Back on my internal medicine rotation, for example, all the residents and the attendings thought that it was quite a good joke to refer to the infamous medical student "sputum rounds" in which we eager-beaver medical students were expected to go from room to room, first thing in the morning, impel as many patients as possible to cough up some mucous, gram stain the mucous, look at it under the microscope, and report back. It is perfectly possible that medical student sputum rounds did at some point or other affect the management of a patient or two, though I can't actually remember that; what I do remember clearly is that sputum rounds were—there is no other word—

disgusting, and that the residents and the attendings enjoyed pointing that out to us and reminiscing about their own student sputum experiences.

And it's another related and rarely spoken truth in pediatrics: just as it's generally easier to deal with children's bodies, it's also generally less unpleasant to deal with their bodily fluids, with their excreta and their mucous and their emesis (though since one of the recurring conversations of our medical student clinical rotations was the question of which is your least favorite, I don't mind admitting that my least favorite has always been emesis). Through the years, as I have practiced primary care pediatrics, I have had many odiferous encounters— carefully preserved diapers brought in by parents and triumphantly produced in their protective baggies—and I never open one of these surprise packages without giving quiet thanks that at least I only have to deal with children.

So if truth #1 was that in internal medicine almost all patients are better left unseen (or at least, unexamined), and truth #2 was that medicine often stinks, we can see that these are revelations actually rooted (no pun intended) in the neurons that make up the sensorium of the doctor. They are not major life truths, though they do, I suppose, reflect a certain harsh corporeal reality: we are bodies, and our precious lives and sensibilities are subject to the vicissitudes and vulnerabilities and indignities that go with flesh and blood. We bleed and we decay and, ultimately, we rot. Or, as Mary McCarthy said in her great essay, "The Fact in Fiction," "You remember how in *The Brothers Karamazov* when Father Zossima dies, his faction . . . expects a miracle: that his body will stay sweet and fresh because he died 'in the odor of sanctity.' But instead he begins to stink. The stink of Father Zossima is the natural, generic smell of the novel" (252). And it is also the natural, generic smell of the ward; the odor of sanctity is rarely to be smelled.

Yes, that's all very well and good, but I can't help feeling that my five transgressive truths reflect something more small-minded and ignoble than the stink of Father Zossima. In struggling with the revulsion occasionally evoked by adult corporeal reality, I was struggling with a failure of empathy, a failure of compassion, and a failure of professionalism. And all I can say in my own defense was that I couldn't help it; and I'm not even sure I get to invoke that defense when it comes to my next truth: the doctors often resent and dislike and even hate the patients.

III. "I WISH SHE WOULD DIE."

The House of God is quite explicit on the subject. Consider two of the laws of the House of God: Law VIII, "They can always hurt you more," and Law IX, "The only good admission is a dead admission" (381). That first law is a locution I remember learning during my internal medicine rotation: there was a lot of talk, every on-call night, about getting hurt by the people in the emergency room, a great deal of disparaging the sieves and admiring the walls, and a tremendous collective hostile resentment toward admissions—toward the feckless ER people who let them through, and toward the patients themselves. We called admissions "hits," and the first question every morning was how many hits the night team had taken—a night with only a few hits was cause for envy and congratulations, while a night with many hits brought on jokes about black clouds.

Oh, yes, they could always hurt you more. It was definitely the ethos of the place, and I am sure I absorbed it from the interns I worked with, though of course, it was only part of their story. What I mean is (and forgive me for not mentioning this sooner), quite a few of the interns I worked with on that rotation were actually wonderful doctors, or, at least, wonderful doctors in the making. They were smart and compassionate and efficient and articulate, and I think they took good care of their patients. But how they filtered that care through the sense of being hurt—and of being hit—I was far too green to understand.

But in addition to the generalized resentment of all admissions, all patients, because they mean more work and less sleep, the narrator of *The House of God* must come to grips with something more pernicious and more particular. "Upstairs, I had just finished working Jimmy over, putting in lines and tubes and starting to treat his untreatable diseases, when Mrs. Risenshein arrested and I was surprised to hear myself cursing under my breath as I resuscitated her, 'I wish she would die so I could just go to sleep,' and I was shocked when I realized that I'd just wished a human being dead so I could go to sleep" (117–18).

If it was shocking to realize that the physical exam could engender disgust, how much more wounding it was to the self-image of a determinedly humanistic and compassionate young physician-in-training to realize that you had begun to regard patients—those wounded frightened human beings who had come to you for help!—as obstacles, annoyances, or, at best, great cases and learning opportunities. You wanted them to stop complaining, you wanted them to stop spiking fevers, and yes, occasionally you even wanted them to hurry up and die. The patients were the hits you took, and the hits hurt you—and they could always hurt you more.

IV. "IT'S MY ADMITTING DAYS THAT KILL ME."

And so no wonder all the doctors were depressed. There's my fourth truth, and I remember coming across it when I read the book after my internal medicine rotation. "During the ten-o'clock meal I asked Fats about Jo. He became somber and said that Jo was terribly depressed. He thought of her as he thought of the Fish and the Leggo and many other Slurpers: terrific medical texts lacking in common sense" (91).

I remember reading that line, and reading other descriptions of the various emotional pathologies that overtake the interns in *The House of God*—the flat affect, the anhedonia, the sense of disconnectedness, and, naturally, the suicidality—and thinking, Of course, that's what it was about that internal medicine rotation—most of the doctors were clinically depressed, and so was I! They were perfectly nice people, they were even admirable people, lured into medicine by a combination of intellectual curiosity and idealism, but they were chronically sleep deprived (this was back before intern work-hour limits, needless to say, in the setting of an every-third-night schedule, and in a hospital where everyone knew that an intern who "called for help"—that is, asked a question—late at night would be regarded as weak). They were tired and anxious, and the emergency room kept hurting them. They were the best and the brightest, but they felt neither best nor bright. That sense of dread that I awoke with in the morning would have been, I suspect, readily recognizable to the house officers—though I don't know that, of course, because we never discussed it.

It is Howie Greenspoon who finally articulates this to the Leggo, who has asked, incredulously, whether it can be true that the interns do not enjoy doing their job: "Y-y-yes, Chief, sir, I'm sorry, but it's true. . . . See, it's my admitting days that kill me. Each admitting day—knowing that the total age of my admissions will be in the four hundreds—I get depressed and I want to kill myself. . . . The truth is, Chief, well . . . well, since September I've been on antidepressants, Elavil" (360).

There it was—Howie Greenspoon was feeling exactly what I had been feeling. He was depressed, and so were they all.

And they had good reason to be depressed. The call schedule was extreme, of course—and it has been modified since, by law. And the ridiculous macho posturing I encountered on the part of some of the hospital staff has probably been modulated over time—I don't know that I believe that a medical student nowadays could be intimidated into administering dilantin by IV push to a very sick patient, as I was, back in 1984. I knew I wasn't supposed to be giving drugs by IV push, especially drugs that the nurse wasn't allowed to give (after all, the nurse knew a hell of a lot more than I did), and I was completely terrified, but I didn't want to be weak (of course, when the patient's blood pressure dropped way down, I got pretty damn scared, and I did call for help, so after that they knew how weak I really was). But I don't think that the chronic sleep deprivation or the chronic terror accounted for the level of chronic depression that I am diagnosing retroactively. I think the depression was linked to my fifth and final truth, the most cosmic and the most distressing of them all.

V. "I HAVEN'T CURED ANYONE YET."

There it is—all the work, all the sleep deprivation, all the depression just circles around the hardest truth of all: these doctors can't cure anyone. Consider Roy Basch's exchange with the Leggo:

> "Well," I said, seeing Dr. Sanders oozing his blood from his nostrils into my lap, "what else can we do? We can't just walk away."
>
> "Right, my boy, right! We cure, do you hear, we cure!"
>
> "Four months here, and I haven't cured anyone yet. And I don't know anyone who's cured anyone yet, either. Best so far is one remission." (163–64)

It comes up again and again in *The House of God:* nobody gets cured. The gomers come in and never die (see Law I of the House of God), and the young come in and they do die—but there is no curing. Or, to let the Fat Man say it: "I'm telling you that the cure is the disease. The main source of illness in this world is the doctor's own illness: his compulsion to try to cure and his fraudulent belief that he can. . . . People expect perfect health. . . . It's our job to tell them that imperfect health is and always has been perfect health, and that most of the things that go wrong with their bodies we can't do much about. So maybe we do make diagnoses; big deal. We hardly ever cure" (193).

No wonder the interns are depressed. No wonder they resent their patients. No wonder they feel repulsed. There is nothing good to balance out all the pain and misery, all the sleep deprivation and anxiety. The patients don't get better. And I have to admit that this is another feeling I remember from academic internal medicine—there were times when it just seemed like no one ever got better. There were lots of grim jokes about the advanced decrepitude and poor baseline quality of life of the patients we often admitted from nursing homes—about the typical patient who hadn't talked in years and hadn't walked in months and was now admitted because he had stopped making urine, so we needed to try to get him back to where he wasn't talking or walking but was at least producing urine. There were jokes about the triumph of the "Harvard death" (with all the fluid and electrolyte lab values absolutely normal, or, as we said, "in the boxes"). And when there was occasionally a patient who could be cured—someone with a bad skin infection, for example, who responded well to antibiotics—there was a real zeal and an eagerness for that sense of having accomplished the holy transaction: patient came to us sick; patient went home cured. But there were in fact so many patients for whom we could do nothing, patients with end-stage renal disease or end-stage cancer, with severe lung disease and pneumonia, with severe inflammatory bowel disease—and then all those nursing home patients, the ones that Dr. Basch and his colleagues would have called, well, you know.

Okay, I have to tell you: I read this over now and I am struck by my own arrogance. Hey, you guys, I seem to be saying, c'mon over here by the pool in Disney World and check out all the cute curable kids here in pediatrics! Look what we have: unblemished and often adorable bodies to examine, poopy diapers that are no worse than what you'll encounter in parenthood, a happy hospital atmosphere with Sesame Street and Dr. Seuss murals on the walls, and rooms and rooms of patients who can be and will be successfully treated! But the truth is, I could be making this pitch, I suspect, from adult primary care or from psychiatry or from surgery. I reread *The House of God*, and I still feel that the take-home message is: Whatever you do, stay out of academic tertiary care internal medicine—and that probably means that I was indeed well advised to make another choice. I don't particularly like or admire my own tone, but it's only fair to point out that in the book's denouement, when Fats and the interns construct a table of NPC (No Patient Care) specialties, they evoke many of the truths I have identified.

Consider the question of the physical exam, for example: one of the advantages they list for psychiatry is "Never touch bodies except in sex-surrogate therapies." And for dermatology, they list "Naked skin—attraction" as an advantage, and "Naked skin—repulsion" as a disadvantage (344–45). Or consider the question of how you feel about your patients—surely addressed by the whole idea of NPC specialties ("PC specialties will not be considered here. The masochists may leave," says Fats [343]). "No live bodies" is one of the advantages of a career in pathology (though, of course, "dead bodies" goes in the disadvantages column). Or consider, above all, the issue of cure, which comes up only once in the whole chart, under the advantages of psychiatry: "Cure—alleged," it says on the list, and an asterisk attributes this possibly foolish claim to Berry, clinical psychologist and psychotherapist and Roy Basch's girlfriend (345).

The lesson that Roy Basch has to learn, in order to save himself, is a career counselor's lesson; he has to switch specialties, to find himself in a world in which he will be able to use his talents and also his compassion. He's made the wrong career decision, and he needs to correct it in order to survive. The lesson that I learned in internal medicine was that I would be a better doctor and a happier doctor if I found another specialty. I hadn't come into the wrong world by going to medical school; I had just gotten off the elevator on the wrong floor, so to speak. I've now been a pediatrician for almost two decades, and I am certainly familiar with some of the awful truths of pediatrics, the ironies and the tragedies. For that matter, I've certainly come across a range of pediatric types who could take their place alongside the savage characterizations in *The House of God*. (Are there occasional self-aggrandizing guys with nonexistent social skills and hypertrophic egos slurping their way through academic pediatrics? Well, sure. They just have cartoon characters printed on their ties instead of subtle geometric prints.)

And yet still, I feel at home in pediatrics. I am happy to examine my patients, and while I wouldn't say that I feel any sense of intellectual excitement when a parent produces a carefully hoarded diaper, I also don't feel any serious sense of repulsion. I generally like my patients, and I don't think that my job leaves me feeling depressed. And, of course, there is the fun of curing patients at least some of the time—or, at least, of watching patients get better. And I don't mean that to sound smug; I mean it, instead, as an example of what we call in pediatrics "goodness of fit," the match between a child's temperament and the demands made on that child.

The narrator of *The House of God* is in the wrong place, doing the wrong job. I reread the book now, and I still identify; I remember pretty vividly what it was like to be there on that tertiary care ward, in the wrong place, doing the wrong job. I reread the book, and I think, thank heavens I matched in pediatrics. Thank heavens I got out of internal medicine, found the right field, the right patients, the right colleagues, the right diseases. I recognize that I have friends and colleagues for whom academic internal medicine provided opportunities for intellectual engagement, compassion, and even curing. It's a question of goodness of fit, and I have no right at all to go around feeling superior, when in fact you could say that what happened to me in internal medicine was that I found myself surrounded by pain and suffering and notably failed to rise to the challenge. Still, there was an important lesson to be learned, a lesson of vocation and inclination. And that's why I read the caustic black humor and the harsh reflections on human mortality in *The House of God*, and I tend to cast it all in terms of vocational counseling and being sure to check the proper box on your forms. There are truths here about life and death and medicine; there are legitimate protests against an inhumane system—but there is also that sense of being in the wrong place, doing the wrong job. And so I am left with the salesman's remark; it's a question, in the end, of finding your right and proper territory.

WORKS CITED

McCarthy, Mary. "The Fact in Fiction." *On the Contrary: Articles of Belief, 1946–1961.* New York: Noonday Press, 1962. 249–70.
Shem, Samuel. *The House of God.* New York: Dell, 2003.

Attending in the House of God

ABIGAIL ZUGER

Around five in the morning you wake briefly then plunge into a terrible dream. You are late, hopelessly, inexplicably late. You are running, teetering in high heels, although you have forgotten to put on any clothes. You realize you are headed for a lecture you never knew you had to give. Then suddenly you are up on stage, naked, microphone in hand, cracking feeble jokes. Then you are awake, too early, for the first day of your last month on the wards.

The hospital laundry room is closed tight, which means you are stuck in a dingy white coat with the dirty ring at the neck. At 9 A.M. you meet your team: two lone interns. Their resident, your deputy, is off today, interviewing for another job. The interns themselves will rotate out of your orbit tomorrow, one headed to dermatology and one to radiology, where they will worry about wrinkles and shadows, respectively. Both are immaculately groomed young women in the latest style of strappy sandal, and both have clearly had enough of the three-dimensional ills of the flesh. They tell you about their patients in lilting, upturned tones punctuated with lots of "no problems." They assure you everything is fine.

You go off to read the charts and see the patients yourself. Nothing is fine. Ten patients, forty problems. Blood specimens taken five days ago from the emaciated woman at the end of the hall are growing bacteria. She has received no antibiotics. She should be dead. As it happens, she is sitting up in bed, slowly eating lunch. The man downstairs who has been in the hospital for four months, experiencing sequential complications of being in the hospital for four months (intravenous line infections, lung infections, leg clots, bedsores), the man the interns told you in chorus was stable beyond stable, has, the nurses murmur, been passing clots of blood from his rectum since yesterday. The paranoid schizophrenic who was discharged six—*six!*—days ago is in bed, sheet pulled resolutely over his head. Awakened, he tells you he is still sick. So he is indeed, sick with his AIDS, his herpes, his anemia, his mental illness; but, alas, he is just not sick enough. He is a little sick: home-in-bed sick, nursing-home sick, outpatient-clinic sick. However, he has no home and will not countenance placement in a residence. Instead, he plans to stay in 9B25, window bed, for the duration. The hospital administration served him with the official final notice of discharge yesterday. He stayed. Last month he was successfully detached from his room only when the city police arrived to drag him away, handcuffed and under arrest for trespass. You try to reason with him. He says he is sick. You say, "Tomorrow." He says, "Tomorrow."

It is tomorrow. The girls in their summer sandals are gone. In their place, you have two new interns: A, a stocky, frazzled woman with a clipboard and an array of colored highlighters stuffed into a pocket, and B, a tall, elegant man dressed in surgical scrubs, with no clipboard and nothing in his pockets. You know immediately that she will be methodical and compulsive, and he will be the reverse. She will worry about everything, even if it is not a problem. He will worry about nothing unless you tell him to, and maybe not even then. Their resident, your new deputy, seems pleasant enough but mumbles so low into his mustache you finally stop asking him to repeat himself.

The bacteremic woman has received antibiotics—A has seen to it. The man downstairs is no longer passing blood—A has everything under control. The discharged man is in his bed, sheet pulled over his head. B shrugs helplessly. The resident has vanished for the day, mumbling about an interview. You call the psychiatrist, the social worker, the chief administrator, and hospital security. I'll go at noon, the patient says. I got till noon. At 2 P.M. he leaves, limping, clothes in a plastic bag, a security guard on his tail. On his way out, he hands you a dense, margin-free handwritten letter detailing his intentions to pursue legal action. At 4 P.M., B happens to come across him lying on a stretcher in the emergency room, bag of clothes in his arms, about to be sent back up to 9B25. He has told the ER doctors he was suddenly taken ill. Unable to find his chart (which is still in a filing cabinet on 9B), they took him at his word. You are a little torn, but B cheerfully upends the patient from his stretcher and walks him out to the ambulance bay, and you never hear from him again.

Every morning there are new patients on your list to meet, examine and review with the interns and resident, and then check on, soothe, and rescue daily until they leave. By rights there should be a flow off that list as well: sick patients are admitted; healed patients leave. This month, however, the earth's gravitational field of illness seems slightly askew. Every day the sick come in, but no one goes home. They are too sick. The man with a fungal infection in his brain will be staying for at least two weeks, wearing sunglasses in his darkened room. The man with an infected heart valve will be getting antibiotics for a month. The huge, silent schizophrenic woman transferred from psychiatry with the third exacerbation of her asthma in less than a month wheezes and wheezes, day after day, long past the time the asthma should have broken.

A young transgender person is admitted to a private room after fainting on the street. He/she has AIDS, and between the AIDS medication and two separate kinds of viral hepatitis, his/her liver is on its last legs. She is actually a lovely, voluptuous young woman, if you don't look too closely. She has been taking a diuretic to slim her grotesquely swollen legs and took three or four or seven or eight more pills than prescribed, just to hurry things up. She wanted to see her ankles again, she says. After a little intravenous fluid overnight, she feels better and wants to go home. Finally! A patient who can go home. She is discharged with good wishes all around.

Everyone else stays firmly put. You haul the asthmatic's old records out of a drawer and discover that she has been on the medical floors eight times in the last five months and has never really stopped wheezing. Perhaps, you think, she doesn't have asthma at all. Perhaps she is wheezing from heart failure or blood clots in her lungs or a cancer choking off the air to her lungs. You tell A to send her off for some tests.

The next morning you hear from a bleary-eyed A—who, in violation of the legal working hours for interns, was in the hospital most of the night—that the patient has been transferred to the intensive care unit. As it turns out, the tests showed she has heart failure *and* blood clots in her lungs *and* a huge cancer wrapped around most of the major pipes bringing air to her lungs. You have hit a trifecta.

Briefly, very briefly, you feel smug and delighted. You have scored a diagnostic coup. You nod sagely at A, smiling at the good news. Good news? You hope you weren't really smiling. The news is hardly good, particularly since it turns out that the patient—still utterly silent, hearing no voices but the ones in her head—has been put on a mechanical ventilator in the course of the night. You know she will never make it off, and she never does. Over the next six weeks, you check on her periodically: she lies motionless in the ICU bed, chemotherapy dripping into a vein, while the ventilator breathes on. Your diagnostic trifecta has done exactly nothing to help her stay in this life or leave it.

New admissions continue to pour in. One of them is all too familiar. Once a voluptuous young man-woman, the person you discharged a week ago is now so swollen she can barely breathe, her skin colored an intense squash-yellow all over from a liver gasping its last. She is twenty-four years old. And she is spitting with fury at you: why, *why* did you discharge her, *why* did you make her go home when you knew she was so sick? She is planning to sue. Her boyfriend arrives with a tiny digital camera to take pictures for legal evidence. He snaps away at her huge yellow legs, abdomen, and face. Then he forgets where he is and lights up a cigarette, harsh words are exchanged with the nurses, and security ushers him off the premises.

Inpatient and outpatient, the impossible dance. By rights, not a single one of the patients on your list should ever go home. They have AIDS, cancer, liver failure, kidney failure. One gust of wind, one cigarette, one beer, one shot of heroin or vigorous shake of the salt cellar, and all is over for them. But the hospital has become a cruelly selective institution of higher healing, and this month you are its designated hitter. You are to take people in, administer a few days of intensive health, and then bat them away. Already, the department is murmuring to you that patients are staying far too long. Your interns have three times as many patients to care for as they should. They have so many patients they can barely talk to any of them; their days are occupied with answering pages and trying to get blood drawn and labs scheduled. And now here, the single patient you sent home (who was delighted to leave, you happen to remember) is sick and suing.

The suit evaporates in short order. She is far too sick to remember anything: too swollen, too incoherent, too sleepy. Her breath smells like a bubbling cauldron of toads and prunes, the sticky sweet "fetor hepaticus" of the dying liver. Her room smells, and all the teddy bears her boyfriend brings in from home in overloaded shopping bags begin to smell too. You leaf through her outpatient chart, a jumble of erratic visits to the clinic for medications to help her sleep, to ease her pain, to organize her thoughts, and, of course, to shape her into a woman until she can afford the final surgeries. Each and every one of the drugs she takes may have pushed her liver over the edge. All of them must be stopped.

But over the course of that first day, an increasingly flushed and sweaty A— highlighters falling out of her pockets, clipboard abandoned on a windowsill somewhere—wages and loses the battle royale of the meds. The dying woman needs them all. She will cry and howl and fling her feces at the walls and torture the nurses beyond all endurance without them. As evening falls, you supervise a compromise, a Geneva agreement of low-dose hormones, narcotics, and sedatives, hoping that somehow all the colorful dimensions of the situation have been made clear enough in the chart that any judge who happens to get involved, whether civil or celestial, will forgive you.

Days pass. It is Sunday. You are where you always are, leaning against the left-hand counter at the nurses' station, writing up the stories of a man who thought he had a touch of the flu (complete renal failure); a man who thought he had a nosebleed (leukemic cells thronging through his bloodstream like spawning salmon); a woman who knew she was dying (everything seems to be checking out fine). A small, smiling woman comes up and asks if you have a moment. She is no older than forty, pretty, curly haired, dressed in some Ralph Lauren suburban line of turtleneck and corduroys that suggests there's a tailgate party and a football game around somewhere. She wants to talk to you about John.

John? Her son, John. She gestures down the hall. You have many names on the cards in your pocket, but no John. You know, she says. Right in there. Oh, you say. You mean . . . Sophia, she says. Sophia, you say. Sophia the yellow and smelly, the indescribably miserable man-woman who is now being dosed with diuretics and cathartics to rid her blood of some of the accumulated poisons her liver can no longer process. In fact, Sophia is actually looking somewhat better, although the room has taken a beating. She is so hugely swollen she can barely turn in bed, let alone climb on a bedpan or other waste disposal device. And no one, but no one, gets to see or touch those genitals, so catheters and diapers are out. Housekeeping is no match for the flow of excrement in that room. A cart with a mop and bucket is now stationed at her doorway full time, but, as the housekeeper is heard to moan after every foray inside, this is crazy.

And now here's Mom, straight from the Yale Bowl. You shake her hand and realize that you have exactly no words with which to open this conversation. Mom goes first. I think he's doing better, she says. I talk to him on the phone every day. Yes, you say, she's a little better. Does Mom understand that "better," in this context, means a few more days or weeks of yellow misery? Even a month would be stretching it. Under other circumstances, John-Sophia would be rushed for an emergency liver transplant, but her out-of-control HIV infection, not to mention miserable track record with medical care, and lack of funds make that alternative impossible.

Mom, as it turns out, understands that and more. Mom understands everything. Mom volunteers in a suburban hospice and understands, among other things, terminal illness, comfort care, and bad smells. Mom understands how to soothe the housekeeper into making another round with the mop, and how to make John-Sophia forgo the jumbo cheeseburger, fries, and cigarettes the boyfriend has smuggled into the room underneath another teddy bear. Mom understands that do-not-resuscitate orders should be discussed sooner rather than later. Mom, who is divorced, has relatively little to say about life in suburban New Jersey with John over the last ten years, a cycle of searching for him in various dives in the city and watching him self-medicate at home. Self-medicate? You know, she says. Heroin. They both finally agreed that John should move out, but they still talk every day by phone. I know I should call him Sophia, she says, but I keep forgetting.

Mom wants to do the DNR formalities before she heads home for the day. You gather the papers and follow her into the room. Hello, my little pumpkin, she says. Hi Mommy, Sophia says. You clear your throat to begin, but Mom is already talking. She gets everything exactly right. She is calm, reassuring. Just in case John gets worse, let's make sure he doesn't wind up stuck forever on a machine. He needs to sign these papers just like Mommy signed hers, just like everyone should sign theirs. The pumpkin starts to cry, stops, starts again, signs. Mommy hands you the papers to sign, and just when you start to think that perhaps this inconceivable Mommy is nothing but a Ralph Lauren–draped automaton, you see the tears in her eyes. You go out to the nursing station and put the papers in the chart and go home and self-medicate with an entire bottle of wine.

For some reason, it is suddenly open season on the liver. Every variety of bruised and dying liver in the city is heading straight into your arms. An illegal immigrant from Senegal is admitted from the clinic, jaundiced and vomiting. His blood tests are frightening, far worse than the pumpkin's. The next morning he is dead, his room empty save for a litter of wrappers and discarded IV tubing from the night crew's efforts to save him. A man lucky enough to have an HIV infection that stays under control without any medication arrives with a liver much like the pumpkin's in happier times. He is just a little yellow, just a little swollen, and heavily under the influence of unknown substances. His sister found him passed out in the bathtub. Soon he is back to normal, snarling that he's not answering any questions because you should mind your own business. He and the pumpkin pass each other on their afternoon strolls in the corridor, nod warily. But this man is on a liver transplant list in Pittsburgh. His sister, elegant in black skirt and silver accessories, visits to emphasize that the transplant people in Pittsburgh must never, ever find out about this episode. It might knock him off the list. You are to write on the discharge form that it was something else, anything else, that brought him in here. The sister's snarl is almost as emphatic as the patient's. You send him home to the elegant Scarsdale home of his elegant sister with a completely unbelievable discharge diagnosis of coma from liver failure.

A weighs the pumpkin daily and points out that if the pumpkin continues to eat potato chips, her ankles will never be seen again. The pumpkin turns to salt-free pickles instead, and the room reeks of vinegar, but ankles begin to peek through. One afternoon the pumpkin proudly, gracefully promenades down the corridor arm in arm with her boyfriend. Two hours later, he is gone, and she is out cold, unarousable. A gives her a little Narcan, a medication that counteracts heroin, and the pumpkin immediately blubbers back to consciousness, cursing and gasping. Another teddy-bear smuggling job. A and Mom have a talk by phone. Mom decides that John is coming home to New Jersey with her once he is ready to leave the hospital. And off they all go, two days later, Mom pushing the pumpkin in a wheelchair, boyfriend following behind with two shopping bags full of teddy bears.

Time winds down. The run on livers ends. A man comes up from the ER, vomiting, with a diagnosis of gastroenteritis. The ER doctor seems to have forgotten to look at his cardiogram. You rub your eyes and look again, and sure enough, he is in the middle of a massive inferior wall heart attack right there in the farthest possible bed from the nursing station. A has trouble finding his blood pressure. Even B stays around late into the afternoon to help. There are no attending cardiologists on the premises any more; they have all been moved to the hospital's Cardiac Center of Excellence uptown. A locates one on the phone and, seven long hours later, personally escorts the man uptown in an ambulance for his emergency catheterization. She states, heading into the elevator, that she has lost count of how many illegal hours she has worked this month.

The interns' last day on the service arrives. A will go off to a well-deserved vacation. B is heading to the outpatient clinics, a big smile on his face. A's beeper sounds during rounds, while B is telling you all about a new patient's infected toe. A goes to answer her call, comes back into the room frowning. B finishes his story. That was the pumpkin's mom, A says. He died last night.

The day passes, and the night, and now it is the last day of the month. A new pair of interns and a new resident wait for you in the conference room, ready to tell you new stories. You listen, then propel them out to the ward ahead of you. They introduce you to a man with explosively bleeding hemorrhoids, a man with a blood clot in his leg, and a woman with a huge liver stuffed with cancer like a bagful of marbles. You shake hands with each patient and ask why they have come to the hospital; you examine them and assure them that all will be done for them that can be done for anyone—given, you say silently to yourself, a propitious phase of the moon, a fleeting half-smile of divine providence, a hardworking intern with highlighters and a clipboard, or whatever it is that seems to allow some people to weather their perilous stay in your land with less damage than others. You shake hands with the house staff, wish them well, and walk away, because it is all over; your month is over, and you are through.

Comments from the
House of Shem

Living with Shem: Reflections on the Journey of a Writer-Healer

JANET SURREY

I have known Stephen Bergman for forty-five years as my friend, life partner, co-parent, coauthor, and co-playwright. I watched him leave Harvard College for Oxford University in 1966 as an aspiring doctor-scientist and return three years later as a creative writer and political activist. I was there through the years of medical school and internship and witnessed the birth of Samuel Shem in 1978 with the publication of *The House of God*. At that time, I became intimately involved with Roy Basch and Sebastiana Strawberry (aka "Berry"), clinical psychologist-in-training, and began living with all these characters. Anyone married to a writer can appreciate the experience of living with the strange concoctions of truth and fiction in characters who overlap but are by no means identical with living persons, including oneself.

I have come not to identify with but to be affectionately related to Berry, the character who both loves and analyzes/interprets Roy through this year of internship at the House of God. In her spirit, I reflect today on this fascinating journey of Bergman and Shem, whose lifework has unfolded to reveal, in hindsight, a unique interplay of writing and healing. The spirit of his writing has always come from the energy to heal and has always been, in the end, in the service of healing, at personal, relational, institutional, and social levels.

As someone so intimately involved with Bergman, and therefore Shem, I believe myself to be one of the greatest authorities on this subject. However, I acknowledge the completely loving, subjective, and biased account of a life partner trying to see or reflect from a deeply interwoven fabric of daily domestic interactions as well as deeply shared life values and work.

WRITING AND HEALING: THE PERSONAL AND INSTITUTIONAL

In addition to *The House of God*, I lived through the writing and publishing of two other Shem novels, *Fine* and *Mount Misery*. I believe these to be the richest and most honest chronicles of the journey of a highly privileged young white man's initiation and socialization into professional training at a particular time in history (1970s–1980s) in the context of the "best" of Western medicine, the

BMS (Best Medical School) and the MBH (Man's Best Hospital). Beyond the learning of the content and scientific practice of medicine, Roy (and Shem) is yearning to learn about healing, what medicine represented to him as a boy watching the town doctor, what Roy calls "being with" patients in a healing, humane, compassionate, and redemptive way. Although there are models and teachers (real and imagined) along the way, including the Fat Man, Berry, and the patient Dr. Sanders, the desire to "be with" is lost and forgotten in the madness of the hospital. At one pregnant moment, as Berry walks away from the relationship, Roy describes his state: "I did not feel sad. I was not tired or mad. I lay on top of my bed and did not sleep. I imagined I felt what the gomers felt: an absence of feeling. I had no idea how bad I might be, but I knew that I could not do what Dr. Sanders had told me to do, to 'be with' others. I could not 'be with' others, for I was somewhere else, in some cold place, insomniac in the midst of dreamers, far far from the land of love" (Shem 317).

In this "cold place," the journey of internship training becomes one of bare survival, accomplished through sarcastic humor, sexual fantasy, contempt, and objectification of patients. During the scene in *The House of God* when Berry actually comes to visit Roy in the hospital at night (this actually happened!) to witness Roy's world, the Fat Man warns Roy that it is impossible for people on the "outside" to ever understand the experience of the real world of the House of God, and it must never be attempted. "You can't use our inside jokes with the ones outside all this, the ones like her. . . . Some things have to be kept private, Basch. You think parents want to hear school teachers making fun of their kids?" (295).

Psychoanalyst Jean Baker Miller, in a paper on "The Construction of Anger in Men and Women," wrote of the portrayal of medical internship in *The House of God* as illustrating "how many emotions—fear, horror, sadness, isolation, and especially pain and hurt—are turned into aggressive actions, even sadism. . . . In such a life course, the participants are taught an angry denial of reality" (5).

The journey of survival for Shem led to this rebellious act of telling the truth as a means of personal healing, and ultimately to the quest for healing the institutions and practices of medicine. Much of Shem's personal journey (from adolescence into adulthood) has been driven by the inquiry into the dimensions of healing through "right relationship," this mystery of "being with."

I have now watched Shem speak at more than fifty medical school commencements and lecture all over the world on "How to Stay Human in Medicine." The paper we wrote together on empathy in the doctor-patient relationship, published in 1994 in a volume on *The Empathic Practitioner,* is a beautiful example of the depth of Steve's evolving understanding of the nuances of healing relationships. Sixteen years after writing *The House of God,* Bergman wrote:

"You cannot be with others' experience unless you are open and touched by others in the truth of your own experience. Mutual empathy, then, is a free flow of shared experience. A person cannot be truly empathic unless s/he has access to his or her own experience" (Surrey and Bergman 129).

And as Chuck, an intern in *The House of God*, put it: "How can we care for patients, man, if'n nobody cares for us?" (400).

In his own journey to "reveal and heal," Shem and *The House of God* have become a beacon for the healing power of authenticity and connections in life and in medicine. Over these thirty years, I have witnessed so many doctors, at every life stage, express their gratitude to Shem for telling their truth, for validating their reality, and for allowing them to feel seen and heard and able to bridge the gap between "inside" and "outside." So many have told him they have given the book to "my girlfriend," "my parents," "my friends," so they will better understand. So many have said how much they appreciate and are inspired and amazed by his courage and audacity to speak the truth in the service and spirit of change.

GENDER AND RELATIONAL HEALING

Shem's third novel, *Mount Misery,* details the insanity of a year of Roy Basch's residency training in psychiatry. This is my favorite novel, because I was there too and shared many painful and outrageous real experiences that took a long time to process and understand. The searing reality of Shem's writing borders on surreal, but from having been at the institution on which it is based, I know the truth of the things that seem most unlikely.

After his residency training, Shem worked as a psychiatrist/therapist for twenty years. He was a committed, caring, and effective therapist and was increasingly authentic and direct in his approach. It was during this period that our work collaboration began. During that time, I was working at the Stone Center at Wellesley College with a group of female colleagues developing a new clinical theory and practice that was eventually named relational cultural theory. This work was built on the pioneering work of Jean Baker Miller, MD, whose book *Toward a New Psychology of Women* (which was published in 1978—the same year as *The House of God*) had shaken the foundations of established clinical-developmental frameworks by critiquing models of "separation-individuation" at the core of human development. Miller saw the highly individualistic Western ideal as more relevant to privileged men's lives in this culture. She described an alternative model of growth within and toward connection as more relevant for women. She described this pathway of growth as undervalued and unrecognized as an alternative to Western ideals of self-sufficiency, independence, emotional control, and even self-actualization.

The relational model posits connection at the core of psychological health, well-being, and growth. Qualities of healthy growth-fostering relationships are described as mutual interactive processes contributing to the growth of all participants simultaneous with the growth of the relationship.

Working within this relational framework, Steve and I in 1985 began to lead what we called "gender dialogue" groups—bringing men and women together in groups to dialogue around gender differences with the expressed purpose of building healthier connections across the gender divide. Over the years we worked with more than 20,000 people in large and small groups, in every kind of setting in the United States and around the world. Steve began to write about his experiences in this context, and in his first Stone Center paper, "Men's Psychological Development: A Relational Perspective," he began to describe the relational disconnections and violations that shape men's experiences in the dominant culture. He wrote about the encouragement of boys and men to separate from relationships in order to grow, and how in "normal" development boys are forced out of open, vulnerable, and deeply intimate ways of "being with" in the name of becoming "men." (How deeply this resonates with Shem's fictional accounts of the destructive and isolating professional medical and psychiatric systems he encountered.) Men, like women, are born with a primary yearning for connection but grow in an environment where male connection is devalued and denied.

Steve and I wrote together of the gender and power constructions of the male-female relationship and then applied this work to couples therapy. In 1998, we published the nonfiction book *We Have to Talk: Healing Dialogues between Women and Men.*

Steve's contributions to the development of relational cultural theory were profound, beginning with his willingness to name the secret truths of men's experience. He wrote about "Male Relational Dread"—the multilayered experience of men when facing women's relational yearnings, the shame, sense of deficiency, anger, withdrawal, and contempt masking feelings of vulnerability, inadequacy, and yearning.

Again, as in his novels, Steve showed the courage to speak the unspeakable, and again, he engendered enormous private appreciation from both men and women, while some (as always with his writing) were made anxious and angry with this public appraisal of male development and replied with stinging critiques. It was in the context of this gender dialogue work that I saw the fullest evolution of Steve as a healer, a writer, and an authentic compassionate human being. Our shared gender journey took us to working with adolescents and children and led to the writing of an educational curriculum: *Making Connections: Building Gender Dialogue and Community in Secondary Schools.*

It is through reflection on the evolution of Shem's work and life that the best appraisal and depth of understanding of the early novels, particularly *The House of God*, can be made

BILL W AND DR. BOB: THE POWER OF HUMAN CONNECTION

After the publication of his second novel, *Fine*, in 1985, Steve began a long period of personal turmoil and reflection about the limitations of a life centered in writing. We began a long relationship with a spiritual teacher and social activist, Vimala Thakar, an Indian woman in the tradition of Ghandi, Vinoba Bhave, and J. Krishnamurti. Her teachings on meditation and the spiritual dimension of life, the application of such teachings to the causes of psychological suffering, and her emphasis on using awareness to work for peace and justice in the world—her challenge to live holistically as a "student of life"—opened up a whole new dimension for both of us to the study of healing and the movement of relationship.

When Steve and I began working together in the 1980s, we decided to work on two projects: one in the area of my expertise and one in his. Through this we could each experience something completely new. In addition to beginning our gender dialogue work, we decided to write a play together about the relationship between the two men—Bill Wilson and Dr. Bob Smith—that led to the founding of Alcoholics Anonymous. From the first day of our work on this play, twenty-one years ago, we envisioned the play set as an AA meeting, the first scene with Bill and Bob standing onstage, speaking to the audience, each beginning to tell his story—about their devastating alcoholic lives, the miraculous story of their meeting, and the beginning of a relationship that became the heart of AA's fellowship and the passing on of the steps of sobriety and recovery, one meeting at a time, and the creation of a fellowship that has touched millions of alcoholics, addicts, and families.

Steve's appreciation of Dr. Bob Smith's contribution as a physician to the creation of AA has been an important element of the play. Dr. Bob's commitment to working with the physical aspects of the disease of alcoholism and his understanding of service to others as fundamental to his own health and recovery were related to his own personal life journey as a wounded healer. This work as much as any other for both of us lifts up the possibility of the movement out of isolation into mutual, authentic human connection generating a sacred, miraculous healing power.

Working on this play together with a vision cocreated in 1986, we went through years of historical and personal research, numerous readings, a small number of productions, and long periods of silence. After nine years resting in the drawer of Steve's desk, the play was discovered for production in Boston at the New Repertory Theatre in 2006, which led to a long run off Broadway starting in 2007. The text was published by Samuel French and produced and distributed as a DVD by Hazelden. Our own journey of holding faith in this work, the challenge of a cocreative partnership, our three-year collaboration with the director Rick Lombardo and the six actors committed to this play, and the thrill of seeing it come to life and touch so many lives has been a deeply significant, life-affirming, and joyful experience.

The journey, profoundly shared, goes on.

WORKS CITED

Bergman, Stephen. "Men's Psychological Development: A Relational Perspective." *Work in Progress* 48. Wellesley, MA: Stone Center Working Paper Series, 1991.

Miller, Jean Baker. "The Construction of Anger in Men and Women." *Work in Progress* 19. Wellesley, MA: Stone Center Working Paper Series, 1982.

Shem, Samuel. *The House of God.* New York: Dell, 1988.

Shem, Samuel, and Janet Surrey. *Making Connections: Building Gender Dialogue and Community in Secondary Schools.* Cambridge, MA: Educators for Social Responsibility, 2007.

———. *We Have to Talk: Healing Dialogues between Men and Women.* New York: Basic Books, 1998.

Surrey, Janet L., and Stephen J. Bergman. "Gender Differences in Relational Development: Implications for Empathy in the Doctor-Patient Relationship." In *The Empathic Practitioner.* Ed. Ellen Singer More and Maureen A. Milligan. New Brunswick, NJ: Rutgers University Press, 1994. 113–31.

Resistance and Healing

SAMUEL SHEM AND STEPHEN BERGMAN

Arts and letters must both reveal and heal.

To reveal means to show the true situation of people and society.

To heal means to show ways to cure them.

THICH NHAT HAHN, *THE SUN MY HEART*

In the autumn of 1975, I stood in the secretary's office of McLean Hospital, a psychiatric hospital where I was in the second year of my residency. The secretary picked up the phone and after a moment said, "It's for you—a Susan Protter?" I didn't recognize the name and, suspicious, asked the secretary to find out who she was. "She says you sent her a novel?" I wracked my brain, not able to recall a novel or her. And then a vague memory of sending off a piece of a novel came back. I had been looking for an agent for my plays and had written her. In a postscript to my letter, I wrote that I also had the start of a novel about a doctor. She had written back that she didn't handle plays, but she would like to see the novel. I had forgotten all about it. I picked up the phone.

"I read your novel and I love it," she said. "You're either a madman or a genius!"

"Well," I said, "I can't help you with that, but you should know that I'm speaking to you from inside a mental hospital at this time."

Thus began the strange and marvelous journey of my first attempt at a novel, *The House of God*. After being rejected by numerous publishers, it was finally accepted by Richard Marek/Putnam in 1977. Just before publication, I met with Richard and with Joyce Engelson, my editor. Naively, I asked if they thought the book would sell.

"No, your book will not sell," Richard said. I was stunned. "Look," he went on. "You've got a lot going for this book—it's about doctors, and that's good, and it's funny and sexy, and that's good; and it's well written, and that's good too."

"So why won't it sell?" I asked.

"Why won't it sell?" he replied. "Because it's a good book!"

This was my introduction to the other side of writing, called publishing, loosely derived, I would think, from "making it public." Over the years and as fiction selling has become a branch of television, I've come to see that writing novels to both reveal and heal has little to do with publishing that writing. I've often been told that *The House of God* would never be published today—"it's too radical." I was lucky in my timing and lucky not just in terms of the novel. I was lucky to have been created by a time that—if you had any heart and soul at all—demanded authenticity and resistance. My core group of interns and I were products of the 1960s, brought up with the idea that if you saw an injustice you could hang together and take action to right it. Witness the civil rights movement and the end of the Vietnam War. We brought that idea into our medical training at Beth Israel Hospital in Boston in 1973, and out of that combustible moment came my motivation to write my first novel.

Not that I was aware of this at the time. Usually it's only later, maybe ten years or so later, that you realize you had no idea of the unseen historical forces shaping you, pushing you one way or another. The core group of my fellow interns and I just did what we did to stick together and stay vital, without awareness of either the source or the importance of it. It wasn't an act of conscience; it was a way to survive. Only many years later, as I was called on to speak up publicly by thousands of medical students and doctors at hundreds of medical schools all over the world, for whom *The House of God* had become a validation of their own experiences and a hope for doing better than they had been done by, did I realize that my motivation had been resistance. Looking back, I now understand that the same motivation has propelled me in everything I've written since.

TO REVEAL: "HEY, WAIT A SECOND!" MOMENTS

"Hey, wait a second!" moments are those times when, during our daily lives, we see something or hear something and find ourselves saying or doing something and we say to ourselves, "Hey, wait a second! I don't want to be saying this or doing this (or doing nothing in response to this), but I am." Each of us has had these moments, times when we let things pass and go on with our lives.

In my internship there were too many of these "Hey, wait a second!" moments to let pass. After going through the experience, I had a clear vision, almost like a voice inside: "Someone has to write about this; it might as well be you." I sat down at first to write as a catharsis, to share with my buddies what had been the worst year of my life. In retrospect, there was a single touch of the Muse on my shoulder, steering me into right practice: *this novel has to ride on humor (much as we interns had ridden along on humor, to get through), or else no one will want to read it.* I sent a piece of it—single spaced, with so many written corrections it was almost unreadable—to Susan Protter, and seven drafts later, in August 1978, it was published. That month of August was the first time in decades that the *New York Times* was on strike, and the novel did not get reviewed there, or in many other places. By word of mouth it started to sell—and then all the hardcover copies were destroyed by a flood of the warehouse in New Jersey. By word of mouth it has made its way in the world. From the responses I have received, I believe its long, full life is because, for the first time in modern medical history, it was able "to show the true situation of people and society" (Hahn 38). Often the truth in the novel was so bizarre that readers must have thought it was a product of my sick mind. Here are a couple of examples of true incidents:

Chief's rounds that day were introduced by the Fish, and the patient was one Moe, a tough truck driver who'd had to wait in the freezing cold during the gas crisis to fill up his rig. He had a rare disease of the blood called cryoglobulinemia, where with cold the blood clots in small vessels, and Moe's big toe had turned as cold and white as a corpse on a slab in the morgue.

"What a great case!" cried the Leggo [chief of medicine]. "Let me ask a few questions."

To the first question, a real toughie he asked Hooper, Hooper said, "I don't know," and so the Leggo answered the toughie himself and gave a little lecture on it. To the next question, not a toughie, to Eddie, Eddie answered, "I don't know." The Leggo gave him the benefit of the doubt and gave a little lecture none of which was news to Eddie or anyone else. . . . The Fish [the chief resident] and the Fat Man [the resident] were getting apprehensive about what we were doing, and the tension rose as the Leggo turned to me and asked me an easy one that any klutz who read *Time* magazine could answer. I paused, knit my brow, and said, "I . . . sir, I just don't know." The Leggo asked, "You say you don't know?"

"No, sir, I don't, and I'm proud to say it."

Startled and troubled, the Leggo said, "In my day, the House of God was the kind of place where on Chief's Rounds the intern would be embarrassed to say, 'I don't know.' What is going on?"

"Well, sir, you see, the Fish said that he wanted the House to be the kind of place where we'd be proud to say 'I don't know,' and, damnit, Chief, we are."

"You are? The Fish said? He . . . never mind. Let's see Moe."

The Chief fairly burned with the excitement of getting at Moe the Toe's toe, and yet at Moe's bedside, for some strange reason he went straight for Moe's liver, poodling around with it sensually. Finally the Leggo went for Moe the Toe's toe, and no one was sure exactly what happened next. The toe was white and cold, and the Leggo, communing with it as if it could tell about all the great dead toes of the past, inspected it, palpated it, pushed it around, and then, bending down, did something to it with his mouth.

Eight of us watched, and there were to be eight different opinions of what the Leggo did with Moe's toe. Some said look, some said blow, some said suck. We watched, amazed, as the Leggo straightened up and, kind of absentmindedly fondling the toe as if it were some newfound friend, asked Moe the Toe how it felt and Moe said, "Hey, not bad, buddy, but while you're at it could you try the same thing a little higher up?" (Shem 244–45)

This actually happened. Looking back, I realized that Hooper and Eddie and I, without knowing it, were using a classic nonviolent resistance technique by saying, "I don't know," when of course we did. We weren't going to play along with the "power over" culture of the House, which we interns often experienced as inhumane and sadistic, and which we came to understand was often blind to the true needs of the patients.

A second scene is more complicated in that it begins in what was "true," what I witnessed, and goes on to what I imagined, to fulfill a writer's desire to move a scene of brutality and inhumanity to one of healing. Late in the internship year I had a patient with metastatic breast cancer whom the surgeons had taken to the operating room, opened up, and then closed again without doing anything—the situation was hopeless. When she came back to the ward, no one had told her anything about what had happened in surgery. I—like Roy Basch—was reluctant to go into her room and made the excuse to my resident that "It's not my job, it's her private doctor's job, or her surgeon's." In reality, that's as far as it went. I believe that one of the nurses finally told her the news. But in the novel, something else happens. The resident, an invented character called the Fat Man, offers to do it. Roy describes the scene from the doorway.

I watched him enter her room and sit on the bed. The woman was forty. Thin and pale, she blended with the sheets. I pictured her spine Xrays: riddled with cancer, a honeycomb of bone. If she moved too suddenly, she'd crack a vertebra, sever her spinal cord, paralyze herself. Her neck brace made her look more stoic than she was. In the midst of her waxy face, her eyes seemed immense. From the corridor I watched her ask Fats her question, and then search him for his answer. When he spoke, her eyes pooled with tears. I saw the Fat Man's hand reach out and, motherly, envelop hers. I couldn't watch. Despairing, I went to bed. . . . [An hour or so later that night] I went back to the ward, and came to the room with Putzel's terminal cancer woman. Fats was still there, playing cards, chatting. As

I passed, something surprising happened in the game, a shout bubbled up, and
both the players burst out laughing. (248, 250)

There was no Fat Man to go into the woman's room. I imagined it all, as a
way to understand what I should have done, what would have been healing,
in that "Hey, wait a second!" moment that I had—to my shame—ignored as a
young doctor and now had a chance to attend to as a young writer. In those days
we were never once taught anything on dealing with a dying patient or giving
bad news. Rather, everyone but a few brave doctors and nurses was complicit
in avoiding meaningful contact with these poor doomed people. In retrospect,
this is why I wrote the scene, to resist the inhumanity shown to those patients.
I started with the fact—my avoidance—then imagined what should have been
done and put it in terms of the imagined Fat Man. In this way the reality of
medical practice can filter into and through creative imagination to fiction and
then, in the reality of the text, serve as a guideline to understanding not only how
things really are but how things should be. This is an example of how to resist
the inhumanity of medical practice through fiction. My guide for this has been
a letter that another doctor-writer, Chekhov, wrote in response to his editor's
unfavorable critique of a story he had submitted, one of the most remarkable
stories in medical literature, "Ward 6": "The best of writers are realistic and
describe life as it is, but because each line is saturated with the consciousness
of its goal, you feel life as it should be in addition to life as it is, and you are
captivated by it."

Life as it should be in addition to life as it is. Without realizing it until many
years later, this would become the motor of my writing.

One final passage from *The House of God* is another "Hey, wait a second!"
moment that, although it showed a limited insight into the year at the time,
took me at least a decade to understand in a more whole way. At the end of the
year, the chief called an emergency B-M Deli lunch to give the interns a chance
to "discuss things."

The Leggo was right: it had been your standard internship year. All across the
country, at emergency lunches, terns were being allowed to be angry, to accuse
and cathart and have no effect at all. Year after year, *in eternam:* cathart, then
take your choice: withdraw into cynicism and find another specialty or profession; or keep on in internal medicine, becoming a Jo, then a Fish, then a Pinkus,
then a Putzel, then a Leggo, each more repressed, shallow, and sadistic than
the one below. Berry was wrong: repression wasn't evil, it was terrific. To stay
in internal medicine, it was a lifesaver. Could any of us have endured the year

in the House of God and somehow, intact, have become that rarity: a human-being doctor? (362–63)

This cycle of abuse—"we went through it, so you have to go through it too"—is summed up by Chuck, the African American intern in the novel, as follows: "How can we care for patients, man, if'n nobody cares for us?" (364).

What I came to understand later is that much of the brutality and inhumanity in the House of God was not about individuals, but about the medical system itself.

The hospitals I trained in and wrote about were large medical hierarchies. In these "power over" systems, someone always has power over you, and you have power over someone else. The pressure of authority—the dominant group—comes down on people from above, and those of the subordinate group tend to scatter. The result is that interns and residents risk getting isolated. They may become isolated from each other, leading to depression and suicide, cruel actions, and insanity. And each may also get *isolated from his or her authentic experience of the medical system itself*—each may start to think "*I* am crazy" rather than "*This* is crazy." This is the same pathological obversion of truth that Joseph Heller so brilliantly described in the ultimate hierarchy, the army at war. The Bush-Cheney regime in America has convinced many of its citizens of the same perversion of experience: "spinning" it from authentic to fear-filled falsity, creating a sense of isolation in citizens that leads to a sense of powerlessness—a position of great use to the government. And isolation—as when an intern like Potts commits suicide—can mean death. The cycle of abuse goes on.

How to heal this? The only real threat to the power of the dominant group—a power that may be based on the hierarchical lines of authority, on race, gender, class, ethnicity, religion, or sexual preference—is the *quality of the connection among the members of the subordinate group.* Isolation is deadly; connection heals. How does this healing take place? By sticking together.

And so, driven by a healthy outrage, in everything I write I have tried to reveal the truth that comes out of these "Hey, wait a second!" moments: in *The House of God,* about medicine; in *Fine,* psychoanalysis; in *Mount Misery,* psychiatry; in *The Spirit of the Place,* the subtle destruction of civil rights and representative democracy by the so-called Reagan Revolution as seen by a small-town doctor; and in my novel in progress, *Cooking for Kissinger,* the insanity of the growth, over the last fifty years, of the American empire—an answer, of sorts, to the manipulative and naive post-9/11 question: "Why do they hate us?" This is also true of two works I've written with my wife, Janet Surrey: the nonfiction book *We Have to Talk: Healing Dialogues between Women and Men* and *Bill W. and Dr. Bob,* our play about the relationship between the two men that led to the founding of Alcoholics Anonymous. The models in fiction and poetry I hold close to me for this lifework are *1984, The Tin Drum, To Kill a Mockingbird, The Quiet American, Uncle Tom's Cabin, The Jungle, The Memory of Fire Trilogy* (Eduardo Galeano), *The President* (Miguel Angel Asturias), all of Gabriel García Márquez, Pablo Neruda, Wallace Stevens, Leo Tolstoy, and Shakespeare. These writers not only reveal but also resist. Not only show what is but show what should be. For millions of us, that resistance is in the spirit of healing.

TO HEAL: HOW TO RESIST

Given my belief in the healing power of resistance, from these thirty years of meeting with medical students and residents, doctors, nurses, and other health workers all over the world from Boston through Berlin to Beijing, I have been encouraged to put out simple ideas about how to resist the inhumanities not only in medicine but in the rest of our lives.

1) Beware of isolation.

Isolation can be deadly; connection heals. Many recent studies have shown the beneficial effects of good connections between caregivers and patients, patients and families, and patients and friends. Much attention is now being paid to things that were once thought "alternative" and that we are starting to describe as part of "the healing environment." Good connection is at the root of it. In every "Hey, wait a second!" moment, seeking out like-minded others and sticking together to take action is essential. Often, if a person feels isolated, taking the smallest first step may be enough: like-minded others will invariably appear, and suddenly there is a group, and then a movement. Nothing is strong enough to resist truth for long. It may take awhile, but as the history of mercenary armies that invade another country—from Ireland to Iraq—shows, there is no mercenary force that can bear to stay longer than the resistance of the natives fighting for their home. History shows that you can't pay soldiers enough to outlast the unpaid souls who demand that you leave—witness the American Revolution. The Roman and the British empires each lasted about 200 years; the empire phase of America (from the Monroe Doctrine, 1823) is now at 185 years and counting.

2) Speak up.

When we notice injustices and cruelties in the medical system, we must speak up. Speaking up is not only necessary to call attention to the wrongs of the system; *speaking up is essential for our survival as human beings.* If we see something and say nothing, we may gradually be torn apart. But large hierarchical systems are expert at retaliation. Speaking up alone is dangerous. We must stick together and speak up *with* others.

3) Resist self-centeredness; learn empathy.

How do we learn to see, in our patients, ourselves? How do we learn in doctor-patient interactions to transform our role from "power over" to "power with"? How do we play our part in those moments that heal—those moments of what Janet Surrey has called "mutual empathy"—when not only do we see the patient clearly and the patient sees us clearly but *each of us senses the other feeling seen?* Those moments in which you can almost hear the "click" of healthy connection? These are the healing moments and not just in my specialty, psychiatry. Think of a surgeon discussing with a patient whether or not the patient should have an operation. In the old days, a paternalistic surgeon might say, "I'm telling you, you need this operation." Lately this has changed to "I've given you all the information, and now *you* have to decide. Get a second opinion, if you like." A few surgeons have gone further toward a more mutual approach, saying, "What are we going to decide to do?" Note that using "we" does not take the decision away from the patient; rather, it lets the patient know that the surgeon is *with* him or her in the decision-making process. Such a statement empowers not only doctor and patient but also *the relationship* between doctor and patient. And if the doctor starts to use the word "we," the patient will start to use the word "we" back. The use of that language will promote a shift to authentic connection, which will ratify the use of the language. It's a miracle of mindful relationship.

How to learn empathy? Try living through suffering with someone—*really* living through suffering—an opportunity we doctors have every day with our patients and, sooner or later, in our "outside" lives. Try life.

I heard a story about a young doctor who chose to work in a leper colony in India. A friend from medical school, a surgeon in Boston, visited her. Seeing her among the lepers, she said, "I couldn't do that for a million dollars!" Her friend replied, "Neither could I."

4) Learn your trade, in the world.

We doctors have to be competent to be compassionate. If we're not panicked about doing a procedure or being with a patient, we will be able to really listen and attend to the person we are with. In addition, we have to be aware of the world surrounding us and our patients. I would guess that we as complicit citizens are causing more cancers than we as doctors are curing—not to mention the latest threats of environmental damage and global warming, drought and flood, moving the flora and fauna in weird directions north and south toward the soggy poles.

That patient of ours is never *only* that patient—that patient is also the spouse, the family, the community, the toxins in the local air, water, and earth, and the world. Medicine is part of life, not vice versa.

. . .

I have been told that *The House of God* has helped to heal some of the inhumanities of modern medical training, and I am thankful for that. What more in medicine is there to resist? While I can no longer speak of the conditions of residency training, I can speak to the most urgent issue in medicine: what needs to be done by us doctors to heal the medical system in America. We doctors are currently working in, and complicit with, a disaster in medical care in America. The current private for-profit system of insurance is worse for doctors, worse for patients, and better only for insurance companies. It is a national disgrace. Politicians in this country, indebted to the insurance industry, use magnificent propaganda to keep the disastrous status quo system in place—failing to fulfill one of the first duties of any government: to provide good health care for all its citizens. In America the propaganda is always the same: call any universal government-run health care system "socialized medicine."

My father-in-law has been battling cancer, and it was impossible and expensive to organize continued care through the private insurance industry. His oncologist prescribed hospice care, and it was astonishing to my wife and me how efficient and comforting it was. Within a day, hospice had a hospital bed in his apartment, three different kinds of oxygen tanks (large and stationary, medium and on wheels, and small for easy carrying), a sophisticated walker with a sit-down attachment, medicines delivered to him at his residence, and, most importantly, nurses and concerned and talented hospice workers who come to the apartment on a regular basis and are on call twenty-four hours a day. The care is not only for those about to die but also palliative care for those like my father-in-law who are dealing with death that will take place at some more distant time. And here's the astonishing part: it is *all free*, paid for by Medicare. Tell this to the opponents of "socialized medicine," especially when they or their loved ones are ill. Why does it work, and why doesn't private health insurance do anything comparable? Because, government run, it is not for profit, and because the administrative cost of the Medicare system is 3 percent, and that of the private health care industry is approximately 30 percent. As I said, a disaster.

This absurdity of health care affects doctors of all ages. Graduating medical students face terms of employment by HMOs that prevent them from taking care of their patients as they would wish. This is our most urgent issue, and one that calls for collective resistance. To address this, I wrote an op-ed piece in the *Boston Globe* describing how to bring universal government-run health care to all of us. I called it "The Doctors Strike" (published under the title "A Strike for Better Health Care"). In it I point out that we doctors are the ones who do the work. I announce a plan to go on strike two years from a given date, unless by that time there is a federal, universal health care system in place.

If we care for our patients and for our Hippocratic ideals, we have no choice but to try. Our efforts, in synch with the rising tide of public and political movements, might just lift us all, leading America into the fold of those rich nations that put first things first: the health security of their citizens. It's just a matter of time.

In response to this argument, politicians will ask, "Where will the money come from?" The question makes us face the fact that we cannot talk about issues in medicine without talking about issues in the larger world. Back in the Reagan era, a famous Harvard Medical School pediatrician named T. Berry Brazelton was trying to improve preventive pediatric medicine, drawing up a carefully structured plan for a day-care/preventive health system to be employed all over America. He came before a joint congressional committee. With some disdain, one of the "anti–socialized medicine" senators asked, "Yes, doctor, and how would you suggest we pay for this?"

"You can pay for the entire system for a year," Dr. Brazelton said, "for the cost of one of your nuclear missiles."

Today, less than one week of the military budget is one *year* of the budget for the National Institutes of Health. What's wrong with this picture?

America, unlike any other Western country, devotes half of its tax dollars to defense. France, which has perhaps the most sophisticated government-run health care system in the world, devotes about 20 percent. The cost of our military empire is the pain and suffering of our children, of us all. You can't practice medicine the way you want to because of the fraying of the fabric of our representative democracy. A little resistance is required.

Learn your trade, *in the world.*

THE JOURNEY OF THE HEALER

Roy G. Basch enters *The House of God* with a wish to become a good doctor. Present with him throughout the year is the Fat Man, the resident, a beacon of hope and healing. Without saying it, Fats shows Roy—and us—that the way to healing is in authentic, empathic connection with the patient, as in the scene with the metastatic cancer patient. This is echoed in Roy's encounter with the African American doctor, Dr. Sanders, who is his patient. At one point Dr. Sanders says, "All you have to do is be with the patient, as you are being with me" (Shem 156). While accepting and using the new technology available in medicine—at its most intense in the medical intensive care unit—both Fats and Sanders are saying, "Don't let the technology make a technician of you; don't let it get between you and the patient. Do what the best of the old docs did—put a hand on a shoulder, show them that you understand what they are going through."

Some readers, both in the medical profession and outside, have called *The House of God* cynical and fatalistic. It is anything but. In fact, if you look carefully, it is redemptive. Throughout the book, right up to the very end, it is crystal clear that there is hope in medicine, as shiny and solid as the chrome of a stethoscope, for doctors and patients alike. The hope lies in learning to *be with* those who ask for our expertise and help—not only our patients but our colleagues, families, and friends. As Roy puts it, in a time of despair, "I could not do what Dr. Sanders had told me to do, to 'be with' others . . . for I was somewhere else, in some cold place, insomniac in the midst of dreamers" (287). Yet the Fat Man's last words to Roy affirm the hope: "But that's the game, isn't it? To find out [if medicine is big enough for you]. To see if it matches our dreams" (372).

Roy leaves his internship year in medicine deciding that the way to learn how to be human, to be with patients and others, is by becoming a psychiatrist. He enters his residency training in a large mental hospital called Mount Misery. Having gone into his medical internship to learn to become a good doctor, his goal in his psychiatric residency is to become a healer. He thinks that psychiatrists will be the most humane doctors. To his surprise and chagrin, he finds that they may be even worse than the doctors in the House. But through another wise resident, a thin, athletic man named Dr. Leonard Malik, he learns to take his understanding another step toward resistance that leads to healing and to a growing awareness. A passage from the end of his year as a psychiatrist shows his realization of what healing is and what part a doctor plays in it.

In this passage, Roy is having a difficult time in a therapy session with a patient he's had the whole year. She is a troubled young woman who has always made him feel inadequate:

> "Terrific," she said to me sarcastically, putting me down. She looked sullenly into her lap.
>
> In the past I might have gotten angry at her, but suddenly I understood. The issue wasn't me, or her, but us. The "we" in the room, which seemed so solid right then that you could shape it, yet so ephemeral that it was the unseen historical forces shaping you. . . . My job right then was to hold this "we," this connection with her, hold it for both of us. That was my job as a doctor. To use my experience with others who had suffered and my vision born of that experience to bring someone who is out on the edge of the so-called "sick" into the current of the human. To take what seems foreign in a person and see it as native. This is healing. This process is what the healing process is. This is what I signed up for, years ago. This is what good doctors do. We are *with* people at crucial moments

of their lives, healing. How hard it had gotten, in these hellish hospitals and institutions encrusted with machines and dessicated hearts and dead souls, to get back to authentic suffering, authentic healing. How much we have lost.

Now I took on the job happily, even with zest. Holding this "us," this connection, right here right now in this suddenly fine moment. Holding this connection as a father learns to hold not so much a crying baby but the connection with a crying baby, a baby overtired and needing to be held and rocked to sleep, a baby who can sense if the arms around her are constricted with anger and trying to control her, or if the arms are open to merely being there with her. If the arms are angry and controlling, the baby will struggle against sleep no matter how tired she is. If the arms are relaxed and open, she will ease down into the featherdown of sleep, yes.

"We've had a hard time, Christine," I said. "Can we try, together, to understand?"

She looked up at me. I sensed her seeing the depth of my concern. I felt that "click" of opening. . . . I saw Christine see it. I sensed her feeling seen. Despite herself, she smiled. We began to talk. (531–32)

Finally, in my own journey of resistance and healing, comes the play *Bill W. and Dr. Bob,* written with my wife, Janet Surrey, and produced off Broadway in 2007. A key moment in the play, during the first meeting between the two men at Stan Hywet Hall in Akron, Ohio, on May 12, 1935, is when Bill Wilson, a stockbroker from New York, tells Bob Smith, a surgeon from Akron, that his doctor in New York City has told him that alcoholism is a disease.

> Bob: A disease? With signs and symptoms, a course and a progression? What, implying what?—a treatment?
> Bill: Makes sense, does it, I mean medically?
> Bob: Yes. Yes, it does. Why couldn't *I* see that?
> Bill: Most doctors can't. (Shem and Surrey 46)

Bob's realization that his drinking—something he had been taught was a moral failure—was, in fact, a disease is one of the things that attracts him to the idea of working with Bill, in Bob's words, "Finding a treatment that we can try on others." But there is a second remarkable realization that Bill shares with Bob:

> Bill: All this time something's been missing. In that hotel lobby yesterday [when I was about to take a drink], I knew—preachers, doctors, my wife, my friends—none of 'em could help me.
> Bob: Yeah, why not?

Bill: *'Cause they're not drunks!* They don't know what it's like to wake up, your head bloody and a golf bag in your arms and a woman standing over you who maybe is your wife—and maybe not—and the veins in your temples pounding on bone. They don't know what it's like, every cell in your body dry as sand, thirsting for the one thing in the world you know will destroy you—

Bob: I do.

Bill: Now I don't want to get too far out here, Bob—we're both men of the world, rational men who've lived through a great war, sensible men—but maybe there's a reason I'm sittin' here. In that hotel lobby, I knew—knew in my guts like a man knows he's gonna die—that to stay out of that bar I needed help. And then I realized that what I needed was another drunk to talk to, just as much as he need me. Friend, I need your help.

Bob: Um . . . how can *I* help?

Bill: I think you just have. (47–48)

This is the remarkable discovery that Bill and Bob made: that telling his story to another drunk could keep a drunk sober. It may or may not help the listener, but it would keep the teller sober. This is not at all obvious and, to my knowledge, had never before in human history been made explicit. "Healing" is in telling about your own suffering to someone who is suffering in a similar way.

In the New York run of the play, we held "talk backs" with audiences. As we listened to their reactions, we came to understand the profound nature of the discovery that these two men made over seventy years ago in a meeting that is replicated every day hundreds of thousands of times, all over the world. In addition to starting a remarkable organization that is nonhierarchical (not power over, but power with) and nonmonetary (supported by passing the hat at meetings), a program that is the most effective long-term treatment for alcoholics yet discovered, Bill and Bob were the forerunners of two essential healing movements in modern medicine. First, they realized that the treatment of the disease of alcoholism had to be what we now call *holistic*—not just physical or psychological or spiritual, but all of those at the same time. Second, by realizing that the essence was a drunk telling his or her story to another drunk, they ushered in the whole "mutual-help" movement—unheard of in medicine in 1935—that now takes for granted the worth of, for example, breast cancer survivors meeting with breast cancer survivors, dialysis patients with dialysis patients, manic-depressives with manic-depressives, and so on. It seems so natural now, yet it never existed, explicitly, before. I firmly believe that it is not coincidence that one of the men was a doctor—in some sense he *had* to be. Later in the play, when Bill gets discouraged that they are having no success getting a third drunk to join them, Bob says to Bill: "I've been thinkin', Bill, about where we've been goin' wrong. We need to find ourselves a steady supply of more *reliable* alcoholics—ones already in the hospital. They always have a batch down at Akron City. What say, Bill?"

And when Bill resists this idea, Bob goes on: "This treatment of ours can't rely on blinding flashes of light, it's about gettin' back to basics—the body, human nature—like the rest of medicine: step by step you try to put the pieces of the puzzle together, until one day the familiar's right there in front of your eyes. Get it?" (73–75).

Here is a doctor who, at age fifty-six, out of the desperate admission that he could not keep himself from dying of alcoholism, realized with Bill's help that staying sober was not an act of willpower or ego but of some power beyond the self. Not God, but beyond self. This I would call the spiritual dimension of healing, which underlies all other dimensions and examples in my writing, both fiction and nonfiction. Moving from "I" to "we." Moving from "you" to "us." Moving from "either/or" to "and."

Dr. Bob and Bill W. stood together in resistance to the medical orthodoxy of the day to heal themselves and millions of others.

We are living in perilous times, as doctors and as people. Our medical system is in shambles. Our democracy has fallen from a shining example of what could be to an obscenely armed empire that is an example of what is, simply, unbridled and spiritless power over others. Hatred is provoking hatred. Our resistance to this is more called for than ever. The key to being able to resist lies within each of us, because resistance is ultimately in the realm of the spirit. As the Bhudda said, in the Dhammapada:

In this world
Hate never yet dispelled hate.
Only love dispels hate.
This is the law,
Ancient and inexhaustible. (Dhammapada 34)

In our current society, where the will of the people is so far removed from the actions of the government as to make it seem that we are no longer living in a representative democracy but rather a military corporatocracy, it is difficult to feel that any act of resistance can have an effect. History argues otherwise. As described above, in 1935 a doctor and a stockbroker were brought together by chance or karma in a tiny room of the gatehouse of a mansion in Akron, Ohio. Both were drunks, the stockbroker white-knuckle sober for five months and one day, and the doctor tormented by a bad case of the shakes from a ferocious bender just the night before. Dr. Bob, dragged along to the meeting by his wife, Anne, told Bill he would stay "fifteen minutes, fifteen minutes *tops.*" They talked for six hours, and they created what might be the most important healing moment in American medical history—they changed the world. They weren't trying to found AA; they were just trying to stay alive. What they were discovering went against every aspect of the prevailing medical expertise. How often is it that we realize later the ways in which "the accepted wisdom" is rarely wise?

You never know where something will lead. When I sat down to write *The House of God,* I was just trying to express something about injustice and inhumanity that I knew to be true. I never imagined getting it published, let alone writing this essay about it thirty years and millions of readers later. The healing essence of fiction is creating a "we" between the author's felt experience and that of the reader. In my fiction, I like to think I am giving readers a sense that I understand and am helping them to both nourish their genius for the real and stay on the side of the angels. I still believe that a piece of fiction written with guts and humor can reveal and heal, making a difference by bringing brutality and hubris to light, and changing things for the better. For every current fascistic act, there is a rising resistance to it. Who would have thought that South Africa would peacefully move from apartheid to freedom—and create the most remarkable of human achievements, a process not of retributive justice but of restorative justice in the service of reconciliation, of healing?

When I spoke to a group of medical students in Berlin soon after the fall of the Wall (another amazing bloodless revolution we could never have imagined), their main question was: "Given the medical authorities, how could you write these books?" My answer: "How could I not?"

In 2007 when Janet and I led a dialogue in Costa Rica between teenage Costa Ricans and teenage Americans, the main question the Costa Ricans had for the Americans was: "What does it feel like to live in a country that's always at war?" The Americans were astonished to learn that Costa Rica, ever since 1949, has been constitutionally forbidden to have an army, to engage in war. They celebrate "End of the Army Day." They are the only country in Central America that has never been invaded by America and are a model of universal health care and education, as well as ecological progress—providing all their energy needs except gasoline from wind, water, and solar.

These two questions—from the Berlin medical students and from the Costa Rican teenagers—are related in the ways I have outlined in this essay, and point a path to our shared endeavor of creating a just and sane health care system, community, and world.

The great themes of fiction are love and death. Death is always a theme in medicine. So too, I would argue, in its many spirits, is love. And one of those spirits is resistance. Love and death. How lucky we are.

WORKS CITED

Bergman, Stephen J. "A Strike for Better Health Care." *Boston Globe* 5 Aug. 2007.
Byron, Thomas. *The Dhammapada, the Sayings of the Buddha.* New York: Bell Tower, 1976.
Chekhov, Anton. Letter to Alexei Suvorin. November 25, 1892. *Chekhov,* H. Troyat. Trans. M. H. Heimm. New York: Dutton, 1986. 167.
Nhat Hahn, Thich. *The Sun My Heart.* Berkeley, CA: Parallax Press, 1988.
Shem, Samuel. *The House of God.* New York: Delta Trade, 2003.
———. *Mount Misery.* New York: Ballantine, 2003.
Shem, Samuel, and Janet Surrey. *Bill W. and Dr. Bob.* New York: S. French, 2007.

Contributors

∼

JULIE M. AULTMAN, PhD, a philosopher and bioethicist by training, is currently assistant professor and coordinator of the bioethics curriculum at Northeastern Ohio Universities Colleges of Medicine (NEOUCOM). She has published and presented her research nationally and internationally. She recently coedited *Professionalism in Medicine: Critical Perspectives* (2006).

JAY BARUCH, MD, lives and works just outside Providence, Rhode Island, where he practices emergency medicine and teaches medical ethics at Brown Medical School. He is the author of *Fourteen Stories: Doctors, Patients and Other Strangers* (2007), a short story collection that won an honorable mention in *ForeWord* magazine's 2007 Book of the Year Awards. His fiction has appeared in *Other Voices, Another Toronto Quarterly, Inkwell, Segue, Ars Medica, Issues Magazine,* the *Salt River Review,* and *Fetishes.*

HOWARD BRODY, MD, PhD, is Director of the Institute for the Medical Humanities at the University of Texas Medical Branch at Galveston. His most recent book is *Hooked: Ethics, the Medical Profession, and the Pharmaceutical Industry* (2007). He is currently working on a book to be titled *The Future of Bioethics.*

STEPHANIE BROWN CLARK, MA, MD, PhD, is associate professor in the Division of Medical Humanities at the University of Rochester Medical Center and course director of medical humanities. She teaches courses in medical history, medicine, and literature to medical students, residents, and faculty at the University of Rochester School of Medicine and Dentistry. She chairs the George W. Corner Society for the History of Medicine, codirects a program in art and medicine, and also directs a dramatic group, Readers' Theatre Players, at the medical center.

DAGAN COPPOCK, MD, served as a Fulbright scholar in Ife, Nigeria, where he studied the divination poetry of Yoruba traditional healers. He received his MD from Yale University School of Medicine. While at Yale, he served as lead poetry editor of *Palimpsest: Yale Literary and Arts Magazine.* He recently completed a residency at Beth Israel Deaconess Medical Center.

JACK COULEHAN, MD, MPH, is professor emeritus of medicine and preventive medicine at Stony Brook University. His essays, stories, and poems appear in medical journals and literary magazines and are frequently anthologized. His most recent books are the fifth edition of *The Medical Interview: Mastering Skills for Clinical Practice* (2005) and *Primary Care: More Poems by Physicians* (2006), which he coedited.

CORTNEY DAVIS, MA, NP, is the author of three poetry collections, most recently *Leopold's Maneuvers,* winner of the Prairie Schooner Poetry Prize. A memoir about her work as a nurse practitioner, *I Knew a Woman: The Experience of the Female Body,* was awarded the Center for the Book's 2002 nonfiction award. She is coeditor of two anthologies of poetry and prose by nurses, *Between the Heartbeats* and *Intensive Care.* The recipient of an NEA Poetry Fellowship and three Connecticut Commission on the Arts Poetry grants, Davis lives in Redding, Connecticut.

THOMAS DUFFY, MD, is a professor of medicine/hematology at Yale University School of Medicine, where he heads the Program for Humanities in Medicine. He is currently a firm chief on the Yale Medical Service and is actively involved in the Yale Bioethics Consortium. He describes medical residency training in "Glory Days, What Price Glory" in *Pharos* (2005).

MARTHA ELKS, MD, PhD, is associate dean for medical education and chair and professor of medical education at Morehouse School of Medicine in Atlanta. Research interests have included fat cell and islet cell metabolism, research and clinical ethics, the physician-patient relationship, and issues in medical education. In her current role, she teaches clinical skills and ethics to medical students in all years of the curriculum and supervises the residency programs.

AMY HADDAD, MSN, PhD, is the director for the Center for Health Policy and Ethics and the Dr. C. C. and Mabel L. Criss Endowed Chair in the Health Sciences at Creighton University. Her publications include numerous journal articles and several books, including *The Health Professional and Patient Interaction* (2007) and *Case Studies in Pharmacy Ethics* (2008), both of which she coauthored. She has published poems in various journals and contributed to the anthologies *The Poetry of Nursing* (2006), *Intensive Care: More Poetry and Prose by Nurses* (2003), and *Between the Heartbeats: Poetry and Prose by Nurses* (1995).

STEVEN E. HYMAN, MD, is professor of neurobiology at Harvard Medical School and provost of Harvard University. He was professor of Psychiatry at Harvard and served as Director of the National Institute of Mental Health. He is a member of the Institute of Medicine and a fellow of the American Academy of Arts and Sciences.

NEETA JAIN, MD, attended college at Stanford University before medical school at the University of Rochester. She completed her chief residency year in June 2008 and works as a primary care internist at Palo Alto Medical Foundation.

She is deputy coeditor of "Reflections," the creative writing section of the *Journal of General Internal Medicine*. She also edited *Body Language: Poems of the Medical Training Experience* (2006).

ANNE HUDSON JONES, PhD, is the Hobby Family Professor in the Medical Humanities and graduate program director in the Institute for the Medical Humanities and the Department of Preventive Medicine and Community Health of the University of Texas Medical Branch at Galveston, where she is also on the faculty of the Graduate School for Biomedical Sciences. She was a founding editor of the journal *Literature and Medicine* (Johns Hopkins University Press) and served on the first Board of Directors of the American Society of Bioethics and Humanities, 1998–2000. She has published extensively in scholarly journals and is also editor of the books *Images of Nurses: Perspectives from Art, History, and Literature* and, with Faith McLellan, *Ethical Issues in Biomedical Publication.*

PERRI KLASS, MD, is medical director and president of the Reach Out and Read National Center and professor of journalism and pediatrics at New York University. She attended Harvard Medical School and completed her residency in pediatrics at Children's Hospital, Boston, and her fellowship in pediatric infectious diseases at Boston City Hospital. She is also an extensively published writer, whose most recent book is *The Mercy Rule.*

SARAH LAPEY, MD, is assistant director for Humanities Education at the Center for Medical Humanities and Ethics at the University of Texas Health Science Center at San Antonio. She graduated from Harvard Medical School in 2000 and completed residency training in the Primary Care/Internal Medicine Program at Brigham and Women's Hospital. She has launched an elective in international medicine, which offers students the opportunity to provide medical care to underrepresented individuals in resource-poor international settings.

KENNETH M. LUDMERER, MD, is an internist, medical educator, and historian of medicine. He is professor of medicine in the School of Medicine and professor of history in the Faculty of Arts and Sciences at Washington University in St. Louis. Dr. Ludmerer is best known for his work in medical education and the history of medicine. His latest book, *Time to Heal* (1999), is an examination of the evolution of American medical education from the turn of the century to the present era of managed care.

SUSAN ONTHANK MATES, MD, has held appointments in medicine (infectious diseases), biochemistry, and literary arts at Brown University. She has published articles in numerous scientific and medical journals, including the *Proceedings of the National Academy of Sciences, Antimicrobial Agents and Chemotherapy,* and the *Annals of Internal Medicine.* Honors for her writing include the Iowa Short Fiction Award (for *The Good Doctor*), a Pushcart Prize, and Yaddo and MacDowell Residences.

JUDITH M. MCCARTER, BA, University of the Witwatersrand, Johannesburg, South Africa, has an extensive background in communications. She worked with Abraham Verghese at the Center for Medical Humanities & Ethics, University of Texas Health Science Center at San Antonio, on a variety of long-range projects.

ISAAC M. T. MWASE, PhD, MDiv, MBA, is an associate professor of philosophy with the Tuskegee University National Center for Bioethics in Research and Health Care. He was recently selected as a Cancer Prevention Fellow with the prestigious NIH/NCI Cancer Prevention Fellowship Program. His research interests include epistemology, research ethics, genetics, neuro-ethics, business ethics, public health ethics, global health justice, and the role of religion in bioethics and public health.

DENIS NOBLE, PhD, FRS, is professor emeritus of cardiovascular physiology at the University of Oxford. His main field of research is the heart, and he was the first to use computer models to understand cardiac rhythm. As secretary-general of the International Union of Physiological Sciences between 1994 and 2001, he played a major role in launching the Human Physiome Project, a systems biological complement to the Human Genome Project. His latest book, *The Music of Life* (2006), is widely acclaimed as the first popular account of systems biology.

ARKO ODERWALD, MD, PhD, is associate professor of medical philosophy and ethics in the Department of Medical Humanities at the Free University Medical Center in Amsterdam. He has published five books in Dutch in the field of literature and medicine about several topics: psychiatry, pain, becoming a doctor, doctors in fiction, and old age. He is editor of the Dutch database for *Literature and Medicine*.

SAMUEL SHEM is the pen name of STEPHEN BERGMAN, MD, PhD, who graduated from Harvard College, Harvard Medical School, and Oxford University as a Rhodes scholar. Bergman served on the faculty of Harvard Medical School for two decades and has published four novels: *The House of God, Fine, Mount Misery,* and *The Spirit of the Place.* With his wife, Janet Surrey, he wrote the off-Broadway play *Bill W. and Dr. Bob,* the nonfiction book *We Have to Talk: Healing Dialogues between Women and Men,* and the curriculum *Making Connections: Building Gender Dialogue and Community in Secondary Schools.*

JANET SURREY, PhD, MEd, is a clinical psychologist and founding scholar of the Jean Baker Miller Training Institute at Wellesley College. She is coauthor of *Women's Growth in Connection, Women's Growth in Diversity, Mothering Against the Odds,* and many other writings on women's relational psychology, addiction, and spirituality. A faculty member of Harvard University for many years, she is now a board member and on faculty at the Institute of Meditation and Psychotherapy in Boston. She is coauthor with Shem/Bergman of a play, *Bill W. and Dr. Bob,* a nonfiction book *We Have to Talk: Healing Dialogues Between Women and Men,* and a curriculum, *Making Connections: Building Gender Dialogue and Community in Secondary Schools.*

JOHN UPDIKE is a freelance writer, and the author of more than fifty books, who resides in Massachusetts. His most recent novel is *The Widows of Eastwick,* out in 2008.

ABRAHAM VERGHESE, MD, is senior associate chair and professor of the theory and practice of medicine in the Department of Internal Medicine at Stanford University. He serves on the board of directors of the American Board of Internal Medicine. His first nonfiction book, *My Own Country,* was a finalist for the National Book Critics Circle Award for 1994 and was made into a movie. He has published extensively in the medical literature, and his writing has appeared in the *New Yorker, Esquire, Granta,* the *Wall Street Journal,* and elsewhere. His first novel, *Cutting for Stone,* will be out February 2009.

GERALD WEISSMANN, MD, is a research professor of medicine (rheumatology) and director of the Biotechnology Study Center at New York University School of Medicine. He has received many national and international awards, including a Guggenheim Fellowship and residencies at the Rockefeller Foundation Study Center at Bellagio. From 1985 to 1992 he was editor-in-chief of *MD Magazine,* and he is now editor-in-chief of the *FASEB Journal.* He is a member of PEN, and his essays and reviews on cultural history have been published in the *New Republic,* the *Partisan Review,* the *New Criterion,* the *London Review of Books,* and the *New York Times Book Review* and have been collected in eight volumes.

MARC ZAFFRAN, MD, has been a general practitioner in France since 1983 and an author under the pen name MARTIN WINCKLER since 1987. He has penned eight novels (including the best-selling *The Case of Dr. Sachs,* 2000) and two dozen nonfiction books on patient-doctor relationships, television drama, comic books, contraception, and patient rights.

ABIGAIL ZUGER, MD, is a physician in New York City and a frequent contributor of essays, reviews, and articles to both medical and lay publications, including the *New England Journal of Medicine* and the science section of the *New York Times.* Her book about the early days of AIDS, *Strong Shadows: Scenes from an Inner City AIDS Clinic,* was published in 1995. She is currently working on an update.